Thai Yoga Therapy
for Your Body Type

Thai Yoga Therapy
for Your Body Type

AN AYURVEDIC TRADITION

Kam Thye Chow
and
Emily Moody

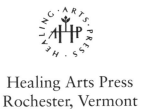

Healing Arts Press
Rochester, Vermont

Healing Arts Press
One Park Street
Rochester, Vermont 05767
www.HealingArtsPress.com

Healing Arts Press is a division of Inner Traditions International

Note to the reader: This book is intended as an informational guide. The remedies, approaches, and techniques described herein are meant to supplement, and not to be a substitute for, professional medical care or treatment. They should not be used to treat a serious ailment without prior consultation with a qualified health-care professional.

Library of Congress Cataloging-in-Publication Data
Chow, Kam Thye.
  Thai yoga therapy for your body type : an ayurvedic tradition / Kam Thye Chow and Emily Moody.
      p. cm.
  ISBN-13: 978-0-89281-184-7 (pbk.)
  ISBN-10: 0-89281-184-6 (pbk.)
  1. Hatha yoga. 2. Medicine, Thai. 3. Medicine, Ayurvedic. I. Moody, Emily. II. Title.
  RA781.7C484 2006
  613.7'046—dc22

                                                                        2006013693

Printed and bound in Canada by Transcontinental Printing

10 9 8 7 6 5 4 3 2 1

Text design and layout by Jonathan Desautels
This book was typeset in Sabon with OptiCivet as the display typeface

Photographs by Ashok Charles
Illustrations and decorative artwork by Kam Thye Chow

To send correspondence to the authors of this book, mail a first-class letter to the authors c/o Inner Traditions • Bear & Company, One Park Street, Rochester, VT 05767, and we will forward the communication.

To my family: Anika, Keanu, and Dana. You are my life, love, and soul.

KAM THYE

For Lila, who continuously teaches us the spirit of play.

EMILY

Love is everything. Freedom is nothing. Between the two my life flows.

NISARGADATTA

Contents

PART 4: A THAI YOGA THERAPY WELLNESS PROGRAM

APPENDICES

Acknowledgments

During my early days as a teacher in New Zealand, a student raised her hand and asked me a very simple but profound question. She asked: "Now that I have learned the massage form, what else is there?"

I contemplated her inquiry for some time. In fact, it was the force that finally urged me to go deep into the roots of Thai Yoga Massage and its well-recognized (although mostly unexplored) connection with Ayurveda, the world's oldest science and healing tradition.

What Ayurveda has to offer Thai Yoga Massage—and vice versa—is profound. Simply stated, Ayurveda provides the Thai Yoga Massage student all of the time-proven knowledge necessary to evolve into a master of the massage. What's more, Ayurveda shows us the way to nurture ourselves and our recipients into a greater state of balance and harmony

What Thai Yoga Massage offers Ayurveda is equally sagacious. Thai Yoga Massage provides an accessible hands-on method for understanding and applying the fundamental principles of the art and science that is Ayurveda and for using those principles for the common good.

These healing methods are linked by a 2500-year-old history. By exploring the historical, theoretical, and practical aspects of this connection, we honor the many masters who have dedicated themselves to putting an end to suffering and to living a life based on the universal principles of truth and harmony. We also help ourselves and the people in our communities to reduce suffering and to realize our greatest aspirations.

I am honored to have the chance to take part in the evolution of Thai Yoga Massage and to contribute to what is clearly a worldwide love affair with and renaissance of this practice. At no other time in history have more people embraced the wisdom, the teachings, and the gifts that the healing traditions of both Thai Yoga Massage and Ayurveda have to offer. I believe we are at the cusp of what I hope is a healing revolution. It is a time when so many people are adopting healthier lifestyles and are gaining a more profound awareness, allowing humanity to identify the causes of illness and to use the tools at our disposal to prevent diseases from developing.

And let us recognize the importance of metta, the spirit of loving compassion that is at the heart of all Eastern medicine. It has been scientifically proven that when kindness is being bestowed, healing powers increase. The purpose here is to live and die with peace, not just to live a long life. Curing disease and unhappiness are not just about treating the body; healing is about embodying the true spirit of love that already exists in and around us.

Personally, I know that life is full of surprises, and unfortunately they are not always pleasant. In the spring of 2003 I received a gift from heaven that I could not refuse. During a Thai Yoga Massage workshop in Montreal, I was diagnosed with stomach cancer and had to have an immediate operation. Of course, this was devastating news for my wife, my family, my students, and my close friends. Facing the possibility of death was the most difficult challenge I had yet encountered in my life. I have two beautiful young children and a lovely wife, who is my angel on earth. During my sickness I was most touched by the outpouring of love from my family, friends, students, and colleagues. In many ways metta has contributed to my full recovery, and life has never been better. I truly believe in this power, and I believe that all the seeds of metta that were planted in my students over the past few years have blossomed into flowers of compassion and were returned to me many times over.

This gift of suffering has given me the opportunity to strengthen my own spiritual practice. I believe that if anyone has the tools to be well prepared for something like facing a devastating cancer, it should be me—although who can prepare for something like this? However, I am thankful for my many years of spiritual cultivation through the practices of meditation, yoga, Thai Yoga Massage, and tai chi. I don't know how people can get through this kind of experience without such support.

I looked straight into the eye of my own mortality. As the Buddha teaches, we are all subject to sickness, old age, and death. In my case this reminder is constantly with me, which makes me thankful for every moment that I have left on this earth.

During my recovery I found great comfort in the wisdom of Ayurveda and used this knowledge to walk the path to full health and balance. Now, more than ever, I respect this healing art.

To my student who first asked "what comes next?" I hope this book helps answer your question.

I would sincerely like to thank Emily Moody, my sister on the path of dharma who had a strong interest in Ayurveda, yoga, and writing. We had an immediate ability to collaborate on writing, and with her help I was able to complete my first book. Shortly afterward Emily's own karma took her to Southeast Asia and India for two years to live in her husband's native land of South India. During that time she studied Ayurveda with the village's Ayurvedic doctor and then went on to study formally with Dr. David Frawley of the American Vedic Institute and with Dr. Vasant Lad of the Ayurvedic Institute.

Since then we have gone on to design the Ayurveda and Thai Yoga Therapy courses and we have taught this workshop both at my school and at Kripalu. Now here we are finally collaborating on this book.

I honor all Thai Massage teachers for their role in expanding the consciousness of this art. Most especially I honor my closest friends and master teachers, Shai Plonski, Paul Cramer, and Blake Martin, whose contributions to this book have been invaluable. I also want to thank my other senior teachers and staff for their inspiration and feedback: Blake, Jyothi, Rishi, Albert, Pierre, Mia, Wendy, Michelle, Devin, Gef, and Suleyka, Csaba, and Tracey. I would like to thank my sister, Poh Ling, for being "Auntie Nanny" to my children and taking care of us in the most challenging time of my life, while this book was also being formed.

Emily and I would like to thank our editor, Susan Davidson, and the staff at Healing Arts Press who over the years have grasped the understanding of our vision intimately and have transformed our words into true art. Emily would like to thank Kam Thye for many meaningful years of friendship and collaboration—you are a true warrior. Thank you also to Emily's brother-in-law, Ashok Charles, who is not only an exceptional photographer but also a joy to work with. Thank you to Catherine Lemercier, Nicole Engelmann, and Shai Plonski for modeling the three main body types.

Emily would also like to thank all the loving hands that took care of her daughter, Lila, while she was working on this book. She is especially grateful to her mother Susan, stepfather Alan, and sister-in-law Gita, who traveled miles and rearranged their schedules. Thank you also to Rami, Uncle Erik, Aunt Heather, and all the other aunties who pitched in—Marianne, Jocelyne, Ilinca, and Ulka. Emily would like to thank her Grandmother Stenger and Mor-Mor Kelly for first setting her on the path of balanced health and well-being. Finally, Emily would like to thank her loving husband, Mohandas, for inspiring her to write this book and for being a pillar of strength, support, and patience. Without you, this would not have been possible.

Finally, to all of our students and to every student of Thai Yoga Massage, Ayurveda, and healthy living, you show us the way for a great today and an even better tomorrow. Om Shanti.

Foreword

Yoga, and its related discipline of Ayurvedic medicine, has a long history as a healing practice. Over time the yoga tradition has impacted much of South Asia, including Thailand, which has embraced many aspects of India's culture through Buddhist and Vedic practices. In each of the cultures into which yoga has been assimilated, it has been the basis of new local developments and insights that add much to the richness of yoga's approach. Thai Yoga is an especially compelling result of this assimilation process.

One of the key concepts of the greater yoga tradition, and a concept central to Ayurvedic medicine and its constitutional types, is the need to adjust the teaching relative to the individual by considering each student's unique nature and the changing conditions of her or his energies, temperament, and capacities. The same practices cannot be given to everyone, and what may be good for one person at one time may not be helpful at another time. Individual adaptation is the key to applying yoga properly.

This need to individualize the practice is even more important when yoga is being applied as part of a healing process, when conditions are yet more variable. Just as a physician cannot recommend the same medicine or therapy to every person or for every disease, neither can the same exercises or set of asanas be expected to work for each person. The individual must always be taken into account and worked with regularly in order to know what will really work, considering who that person is as well as the condition of the body and environment.

Though they have their specific structural effects, yogic asanas can be varied in terms of their energies. Pranayamas are more fixed in their energies, but they too can be varied in their effects according to the way in which they are performed. Individualizing treatment is not just a mechanical issue of applying one asana or practice; it requires working with the person in terms of attitude, energy, and awareness, as well as according to the specific procedures that may be recommended, considering that individual's body, mind, and spirit.

According to Ayurvedic medicine, asana is an ideal therapy for musculoskeletal disorders, whether the condition is owing to internal organic factors or external structural problems. Combined with massage by a healer in whom the prana, or inner life-force, is awakened, yoga asanas have yet more power. Ayurveda considers pranayama to be the ideal tool for balancing the doshas at an organic level, helping us to adjust the prana that is behind all three doshas of vata (air), pitta (fire), and kapha (water). Pranayama is an important part of all therapies and of any healthy lifestyle.

Thai Yoga Therapy for Your Body Type is unique in that it brings together these key concepts of yoga and Ayurveda for determining individual type and condition. This adds a great deal of depth and specificity to the treatment. The authors link yoga therapy with the broader range of Ayurvedic lifestyle recommendations relative to individual constitution; those recommendations include diet, which is central to how the physical body functions and moves. This range of treatment recommendations places yoga therapy in the context of an entire set of natural healing practices, providing the opportunity for yoga to impact the whole of our lives.

The authors look at yoga asanas as part of this greater system of Ayurvedic healing, providing guidance through which the asanas can be more effectively utilized. For the reader unfamiliar with these concepts, *Thai Yoga Therapy for Your Body Type* explains the three doshic types of vata, pitta, and kapha in clear terms. The text examines the role of the five vayus (prana, apana, samana, udana, and vyana) and their energetic effects, important for determining the effects of asanas and pranayamas. They consider not only the condition of the physical body but all of the five koshas, or sheaths of the soul, which reflect the deeper levels of our being.

The book is practical, providing many specific and well-delineated exercises that can be useful for a broad range of health conditions. The authors have condensed a great deal of important information in this single volume, reflecting much experience and insight from their own work and study.

I have personally met Kam Thye Chow and Emily Moody, and was I impressed by their degree of insight and willingness both to look into the Ayurvedic roots of Thai Yoga Therapy and to develop those connections further in light of current knowledge. Their book is a welcome contribution to the field and helps open the way for further research and examination. I have also experienced the authors' treatment methods.

Thai Yoga massage is a gentle, relaxing form of treatment that stimulates the higher sattvic (spiritual) vibrations of the mind and heart. It is useful for health maintenance as well as for treating a variety of conditions.

When yoga therapy is employed according to non-yogic systems of medicine, asanas often get reduced to a mere adjunct or technique of physical therapy, which is the case for much of yoga therapy today. Ayurveda helps restore yogic healing to its real breadth and depth. Ayurvedic medicine provides us with a complete yogic system of medicine in terms of philosophy, diagnosis, and treatment methods. It forms the ideal foundation for the application of yoga therapy as well as offering the appropriate support practices of diet, herbs, massage, and other clinical procedures to link it to the whole of medical practice.

It is important that all yoga therapists consider the role of Ayurveda in yoga therapy and learn to benefit from its many tools of health, well-being, and inner transformation. The authors have shown how to bring an Ayurvedic perspective into Thai Yoga Therapy, which greatly enhances this system of healing. The book is an important addition to the literature on yogic healing. It is hoped that more yoga teachers will take such an approach in their work and studies. It is also an important book for Ayurvedic students, relative to both yoga and massage, and adds many new insights for their work as well.

Dr. David Frawley
Author of *Yoga and Ayurveda, Yoga for Your Type,* and
Ayurveda and Marma Therapy
Director of the American Institute of Vedic Studies

PART 1

❖❖

The Ayurvedic Foundations of Thai Yoga Therapy

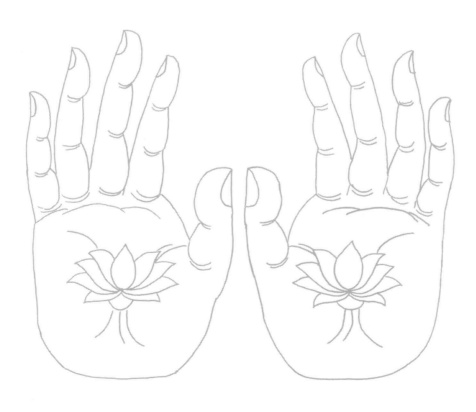

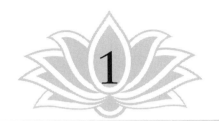

The Buddha's Medicine Travels to Thailand

In Thailand there is a legendary tale about a group of monks who relocated a large clay Buddha in Bangkok. To the great horror of the monks, the giant idol was accidentally dropped during the move and came crashing loudly to the ground. When the head monk returned later that night to inspect the damage, he noticed a crack in the side of the statue. As he shined his flashlight on the damaged area, the monk was startled to see a bright reflection gleaming out of the crack. Using a chisel and hammer, the curious monk began to chip away at the clay; with each chip the gleam grew brighter and bigger.

After hours of labor the monk found himself face to face with a glimmering Buddha made of solid gold. Following an investigation it was discovered that the treasure had been camouflaged in clay during the Burmese invasions to disguise its significant value. The golden Buddha now resides in Bangkok in Wat Traimit, the Temple of the Golden Buddha.

Like this golden Buddha, each and every one of us has an inner beauty of infinite value. Revealing the golden Buddha nature within is the true purpose of both Ayurveda and Thai Yoga Therapy, sister sciences in the venerable traditions of the East.

Ayurveda and Thai Yoga Therapy share a common historical lineage that dates back to the beginnings of Vedic philosophy some five thousand years ago. At around this time the guiding principles of Ayurveda and the entire Vedic system were revealed to the great sages of ancient India. From these insights came a profound theory of creation known as Samkhya philosophy, which is the base of Ayurveda, yoga, and Thai Yoga Massage.

According to this theory, the universe is created through a cause-and-effect exchange between two primary forces: Purusha, or unmanifested energy, and Prakruti, or matter. Purusha is pure consciousness that witnesses the act of creation, while Prakruti is the feminine energy that makes all creation possible.

Out of the celestial dance between these forces comes the collective form of cosmic intelligence known as Mahad. The moment the understanding of self is differentiated from the collective intelligence of Mahad, the ego of Ahamkara is born. The concept of "I" emerges as the individual self becomes the center of consciousness.

Samkya Creation Philosophy

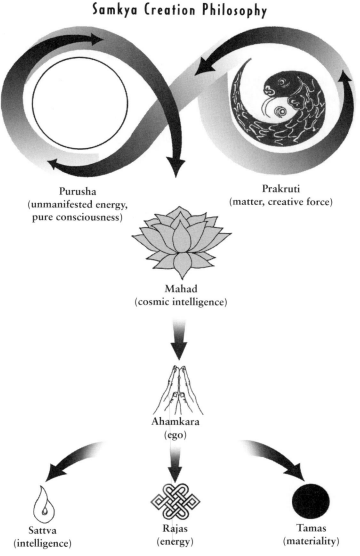

Samkhya philosophy, the theoretical foundation of Ayurveda, yoga, and Thai Yoga Massage, contemplates the journey of consciousness into matter.

It is only through the ego that the three creative forces of the gunas can be perceived and experienced. Each physical manifestation that we experience in our everyday lives is composed of some combination of the three gunas: *sattva, rajas,* and *tamas.* The *sattva guna* is the subtle energy of cognition that forms the mind, the senses, and the motor pathways of the body. The *tamas guna* is the gross force that creates the five great elements of earth, air, fire, water, and ether, and the *rajas guna* is the vital force that activates the other two gunas.

The concept of truth, or *san,* is at the core of Samkhya philosophy. Each step along the path of self-awareness brings us closer to being reunited with the divine consciousness of the universe, to experiencing the full potential of our being in this lifetime. As we better understand the Samkhya concept of truth in our daily lives, we begin to observe the interconnectedness of all beings. This is particularly important to our work as healers. The less entrenched we are in the ego of Ahamkara, for example, the more we can focus on the true needs, concerns, and dreams of those around us. When we connect with the divine intelligence of Mahad, our lives and healing practices become full of compassion and loving-kindness.

The aim of Ayurveda is to reveal the true nature of oneself, not only in terms of our particular body type, but as interconnected with the overall divine consciousness of the universe.

The comprehensive medical system known as Ayurveda has been practiced in India for several centuries. The word Ayurveda literally means "the science of life" (*ayur,* "life," and *veda,* "science"). This ancient system offers a sophisticated understanding of preventive health practices and long-term wellness based on an individualized approach to body types.

The first written record of Ayurveda can be found in the *Rig Veda* (c. 3000 BCE), the most ancient of the four scriptures that form the backbone of Vedic philosophy. The oldest known song in the world, the *Rig Veda* describes the medicinal uses of many Ayurvedic herbs and mantras. This volume speaks of three main Ayurvedic "powers," the first reference to the principle of the three doshas of *vata, pitta,* and *kapha.* The fourth Veda, *Artharva Veda,* dates back to around 2000 BCE and contains the most detailed information on Ayurveda, with instruction in the use of mantras, medicinal plants, and therapeutic gems. Within the discipline of Ayurveda, the *Artharva Veda* is known as the most crucial of the four Vedas, as it contains direct information pertaining to the practice of Ayurveda.

Several important treatises appeared between 400 BCE and 500 AD to form the basis of modern-day Ayurveda. The most celebrated works from this period were written by the three great Ayurvedic physicians Charaka, Sushruta, and Vagbhatta. Charaka composed the first of these texts, *Charaka Samhita,* which is widely acknowledged as the basis of modern Ayurveda. Still used extensively, this voluminous work concentrates on internal medicine and the use of diet and herbs for healing. *Sushruta Samhita*, titled after the great Ayurvedic physician Sushruta, appeared several decades later and focuses on the practice of Ayurvedic surgery. *Astanga Hridaya*, the third of the great classical texts, was written by Vagbhatta as a concise compilation of the two earlier texts. These three works remain the primary textbooks for Ayurvedic study in India to the present day.

During the third century BCE, Ayurveda experienced a period of vitalization under the leadership of Emperor Ashoka. Ashoka was a famous Hindu warrior who renounced violence for the teachings of the Buddha and opened the way for the proliferation of Buddhism throughout Southeast Asia. Central to the Buddha's teachings is the alleviation of all suffering, including physical illness. When the Buddhist monks migrated overseas to export the teachings of the Buddha, their Ayurvedic medical practices went with them. Ayurveda subsequently became an established healing practice in the countries of Sri Lanka, Thailand, and Burma as Buddhism spread throughout the East.

The medicinal system of Ayurveda laid the foundation for many highly respected Eastern healing practices. The relationship between Ayurveda and Thai Yoga Massage dates back to the fifth century BCE in India, during the time of the Buddha. A famous story from this period tells of a student in northern India who was given a final question as part of his examination to become an Ayurvedic physician. Five graduating students were asked to roam within a few miles' radius of the school and to come back with a product of nature void of any medicinal value. The students returned, one by one, and each presented his findings—a human skull, poison, a rock, and a fish carcass. After some time the fifth student returned, declaring, "Sir, I cannot find anything that is not of medicinal value!" Everything that he encountered in the forest, to his thinking, had some therapeutic value. It was only this student who passed the exam, illustrating the Ayurvedic principle that everything around us can and should be used for healing purposes.

The illustrious student in this anecdote was Jivaka Kumarbhaccha, who went on to become the venerated physician to the Buddha and the founding father of the healing art of Thai Yoga Massage. Jivaka was born some time around the fifth century BCE and was said to have been abandoned by his mother, who placed the newborn infant in a wooden box in a rubbish heap beside the road. Later that same day Prince Abhaya, a son of King Bimbisara, discovered the baby and, moved by compassion, decided to raise Jivaka as his adopted son. It was through this fortunate event that Jivaka grew to become a famous royal physician in the court of Bimbisara of Magadha, whose kingdom was in northern India.

Tales about Jivaka's medical feats and cures can be found in almost all versions of Buddhist scripture. He was so renowned that many joined the Buddhist community in Magadha just to be availed of his teachings. Although Jivaka never actually traveled to

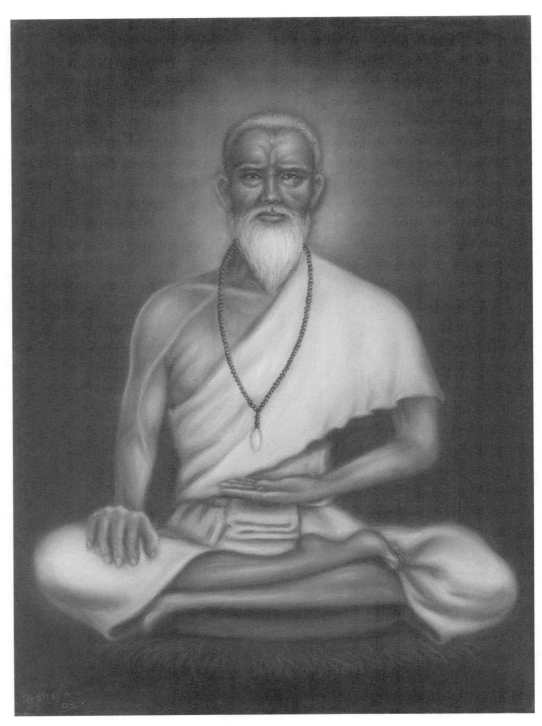

Jivaka Kumarbhaccha, the founding father of Thai massage and Thai Ayurveda

Thailand, his teachings became the foundation of traditional Thai massage when they were transported to Southeast Asia with the spread of Buddhist Indian culture. In many temples throughout Thailand, a shrine is dedicated to Jivaka as a central figure in Thai medical and traditional massage practices. Thai massage healers often open the day with a chant in honor of Jivaka to draw insight from his healing spirit.

Over the centuries Ayurveda has assimilated into the predominant Thai culture, evolving into a distinctive folk medicine. Traditional Thai massage, or *nuad boran*, is often used in combination with Ayurvedic herbal steam baths, hot compresses, and herbal concoctions. Many practitioners of traditional Thai medicine may not actually use the term Ayurveda in defining their work, but the connection to this ancient system is clearly evident in their practices and nomenclature.

Similar to its Indian predecessor, Thai Ayurveda focuses on the circulation of prana, the vital energy that makes all life possible. Pranic energy—or *lom pran,* as it is called in Thai—is key to achieving optimal balance and health according to both systems. Thai and Indian Ayurveda are both based on the elements theory and share common linguistic references in this regard. For example, the Thai terms *vayo* (wind) and *apo* (water) can be compared to the Sanskrit words *vayu* and *apas* of the same meaning. Another interesting connection between the healing traditions of India and Thailand is the practice of *ruesri dut ton,* a form of yoga that developed in Thailand many centuries ago. It is believed that this system was developed by the religious Thai hermits known as the *ruesris,* whose title bears a striking resemblance to the prophetic *rishis* of India.

Through the generations Thai Ayurveda has been orally passed down as a folk medicine in villages across Thailand. In contrast to its Indian counterpart, there is little written documentation of the historic development of Ayurveda in Thailand. Furthermore, due to the prevalence of Chinese culture and a native village shamanic practice within Thailand, Thai Ayurveda has taken on an ecumenical flavor of its own. A unique folk medicine that is indigenous to Thailand has resulted.

Through time the science and practice of traditional Indian Ayurveda in Thailand has been diluted, reduced to mostly pharmaceutical purposes, with little reference to its profound theoretical foundations. However, more recently Thai Ayurveda has experienced renewed interest and is beginning to appear in modern facilities such as the Phuket Hospital in southern Thailand and in health spas and tourist sites. The Thai health community is expressing a growing desire to reconnect with Ayurveda and several organizations have been established for this specific purpose. With the rapidly growing popularity of Thai massage in Thailand and around the world, many students and practitioners seek a deeper understanding of the therapeutic roots underlying this dynamic and effective massage form.

The method of bodywork that we have developed, Lotus Palm Thai Yoga Therapy, is so named for the integration of Thai Yoga Massage with its ancient Ayurvedic roots.

For many, Ayurveda can be highly conceptual and sometimes hard to grasp, yet when experienced firsthand through the physical body, this profound science is grounded and more easily digested. Each Thai Yoga Therapy session becomes a customized treatment tailored to a person's unique Ayurvedic body type; in this way, Thai massage is transformed into a vehicle for channeling the foundational wisdom of Ayurveda. Using an Ayurvedic constitutional assessment and designing follow-up sessions in concert with the client, the therapist learns more about each client. A stronger client-therapist alliance is formed, encouraging greater healing potential.

The founding father of Thai Yoga Massage dedicated his life to healing others through Ayurveda, massage, and the Buddhist virtues of loving-kindness and compassion. By reuniting traditional Ayurveda and Thai Yoga Massage, we hope to bring out the depth of healing potential unveiled centuries ago by Jivaka. May you carry these teachings in the spirit of divine connection and humble gratitude with which they are shared.

Ayurveda and the Five Elements of Life

According to Ayurveda, the natural system of balance that rules the cosmos is at play within the human body and mind. When we allow our inner nature to govern our choices and lifestyle and acknowledge any imbalances that do arise, a sense of positive functioning and equilibrium naturally follows. If, on the other hand, we are ruled by external influences and continuously ignore the natural needs of our body, imbalances and disease are certain to occur. Every day, when we choose a certain food, lifestyle habit, or exercise, nature sends us messages about the soundness of our decision. For example, some individuals experience an acidic reaction in the stomach after eating spicy foods or tomatoes; this is the body's way of saying that a different food choice would be more suitable. A common response is to ignore such messages, or to mask the symptoms (by digesting an antacid tablet, in this instance). But by ignoring the sophisticated feedback system of the body we override our inner wisdom and become vulnerable to developing serious conditions such as heartburn or stomach ulcers.

Every day we are faced with a series of choices: what to eat, what exercise to engage in, how to use our free time, which habits to maintain or abandon. Each of these individual choices has the potential to create balance or cause imbalance, depending on each person's unique constitution. With Ayurveda at the base, the Thai Yoga Therapy practitioner can help clients reach a higher state of harmony by fusing body movement and breathwork with a balanced approach to everyday living. As we focus through the lens of Ayurveda we are provided with a beautiful insight into the nature of the universe, beginning with the five great elements.

THE GREAT ELEMENTS

According to Ayurveda, everything in the universe is composed of the five elements, or *panchamahabhutas*. The elements of earth, water, fire, air, and ether are present in all matter, including our own physical and mental bodies. The way in which these elements combine in our bodies is one of the factors contributing to our uniqueness, our Ayurvedic "fingerprint."

Let's consider a few easy examples of ways in which the elements show as tendencies in a person's body and nature. Take, for instance, a person with a high proportion of earth in his or her constitution. Such a person may be grounded and "down to earth" but could also be prone to stagnation and slow to change. A person with a high level of air may be very creative but may be prone to "spacey-ness" or nervousness. The absence of certain elements also expresses itself in the body and mind. For example, a person with a low level of the fire element may tend to be cold and have a weak digestive fire; on a mental level he or she may experience a lack of passion for life.

The elements theory is the fundamental basis of many Eastern philosophies, with slight variations from region to region. In Thailand, a four-element system is practiced based on earth *(pattavee)*, wind *(vayo)*, fire *(taecho)*, and water *(apo)*. In exploring the traditional Ayurvedic underpinnings to Thai Yoga Therapy, however, we will address all five elements in our discussion here.

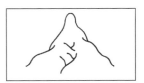

Earth provides the structure for all animate and inanimate objects in the universe. In nature it is found in the substances of rock and soil, which provide a stable foundation for roots to form and grow. Within the body, earth forms the skeletal system, tissues, cells, and the overall physical form. In Ayurveda, earth represents steadiness, static energy, and groundedness.

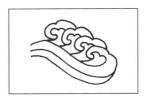

Water represents the flowing motion that nurtures and sustains life. It exists in the moving cycle of precipitation that begins with evaporation, forms into clouds, and finally returns as rain; water can be found in the icy snowcaps of a mountain and the flowing river meandering down to the open sea. In the body, water is the movement of blood, lymph, and liquid matter. This cycle of movement keeps the body healthy by eliminating waste products and circulating nutrients. In Ayurveda, water symbolizes emotion, vitality, and life.

Fire is the source of all physical and mental transformation in the body. It is responsible for the combustion of solid to liquid and liquid to gas. In nature, the fire of the sun governs the processes of creation and destruction of all life forms. In the body, fire governs the process of digestion and metabolism as well as all forms of perceiving and processing on the mental plane.

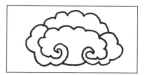

Air is the life force that moves all bodily systems, thoughts, and ideas. This element enables the qualities of creativity and adaptability to exist. In nature, air is found in the oxygen we breathe and in the wind blowing through the trees. Within the body, air governs coordination, the nervous system, and the respiratory system as well as creative thinking. In Ayurveda, air represents movement, change, and tolerance.

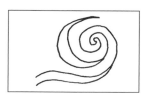

Ether is the most subtle of all the elements and provides the space for all the other elements to exist. It maintains space between objects, which allows for distinction between forms. Within nature, ether is the gaseous substance that creates cloud formations and the earth's atmosphere. In the body ether corresponds to the spaces within the pelvic cavity, mouth, ears, nostrils, abdomen, and respiratory tract. Ether governs the sense of sound and represents consciousness, inner knowledge, and peace.

THE TRIDOSHAS

According to Ayurveda, the five great elements combine to form three vital forces that are present in everybody and everything. These three forces are known in Sanskrit as the *tridoshas*, or "three doshas," of vata, pitta, and kapha.

All the physiological and psychological processes that enable human existence are governed by the doshas. When in balance, the doshas maintain a state of equilibrium and bring us vigor, longevity, and an overall state of well-being. When out of balance they become the agents of impurity and disease.

One of the easiest ways to understand the doshas is to consider the predominant elements that make up each doshic force. As depicted on the following page, vata is formed by the primary element of air and secondary element of ether; pitta is formed by the primary element of fire and secondary element of water; and kapha consists of water and earth, with water predominating.

As our understanding of Ayurveda deepens and we begin to apply the concepts of

The Ayurvedic Doshas

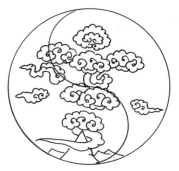

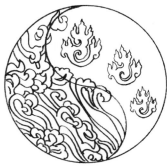

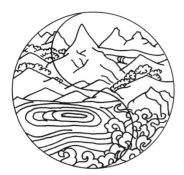

Vata (air + ether):   Pitta (fire + water):   Kapha (water + earth):
nervousness   passion   inactivity

the tridoshas, it is useful to continuously refer back to the primary and secondary elements of each dosha. This provides a reminder that we are essentially working on the elements at play within each client's body. (The Buddha is quoted to have once said, "You are not the elements that make up the body, you are that which makes use of the elements.") Some Ayurvedic scholars refer to the doshas and the primary element as one and the same, describing vata as "air," pitta as "fire," and kapha as "water." However, consideration of the secondary element is essential to our understanding of the dynamic interplay between elements that make up each unique body.

In considering the relationship between the primary and the secondary elements in a given dosha, it is helpful to consider the analogy developed by Dr. Vasant Lad. Dr. Lad imagines the secondary element of a dosha to be a clay pot that functions as a container for carrying the "content" of the primary element. For kapha, then, the primary element of water is carried by earth, the secondary element. This relationship parallels those found in the body as well. For example, the kaphic fluid of phlegm consists of the primary element of water as the content and the secondary element of earth as the container.

Anatomically speaking, each of the doshas is responsible for different functions within the body. Similar to the function of wind in nature, the vata dosha governs all bodily movement. On a physical level this corresponds to motor function, limb coordination, circulation, respiration, digestion, and elimination. On a mental level vata governs the movement of thoughts, feelings, and nerve impulses, allowing for communication and creativity to occur. A healthy functioning of vata leads to an efficient and smooth flow along these channels, while an unhealthy functioning of vata causes obstructions, stagnation, and irregular movement.

The pitta dosha can be imagined as a flame that enlivens all bodily processes of digestion. Pitta governs the absorption of all foods and liquids and is responsible for metabolism and absorption, and for maintaining the appetite, body temperature, and eyesight. The pitta flame is also present in the mind, where all thoughts and ideas are digested, leading to intelligence, clarity, and perception.

The kapha dosha is related to nourishment and stability within the body. Kapha provides the overall structure of the body, giving shape and form to bones, tissues, and organs. It also governs lubrication, fat regulation, sleep, energy, and stamina and is responsible for maintaining all bodily fluids. Mentally, kapha brings stability, contentment, forgiveness, groundedness, and compassion.

The doshas coexist in a symbiotic relationship within the body and share an equally important role in the creation and sustenance of life. Just as nature cannot exist without the elements of air, fire, and water, each individual body cannot operate without the presence of vata, pitta, and kapha. When a Thai Yoga Therapy practitioner is able to recognize the constitutional differences between each recipient, as evidenced by the doshas, a customized approach based on individual qualities and needs unfolds. A massage approach that is good for one individual may not be good for another. What may calm and restore a hyperactive vata person may cause a kapha person to become sleepy and sluggish. The stimulating approach that invigorates and energizes kapha people may overheat pitta individuals, leaving them red in the face and even agitated by a massage.

Through the looking glass of Ayurveda we begin to see distinctions that are often overlooked in a more standardized approach to massage and bodywork. In Thai Yoga Therapy we encourage clients to become self-educated about the interplay of the elements in their bodies by inviting them to fill out an Ayurvedic constitutional test, which you will find in the appendix. This test assists both client and practitioner in addressing the body's needs. When a session is individually tailored, clients walk away from a massage with a greater sense of satisfaction and rejuvenation. In addition to providing a customized bodywork session, Thai Yoga Therapy practitioners have the opportunity to introduce the powerful system of Ayurveda to clients in a noninvasive and easy-to-follow format. With each session we plant the seeds of Ayurveda into the minds and hearts of our clients, and those seeds are likely to blossom for many years to come.

ASSESSING THE DOSHIC CONSTITUTION

During the process of human conception the forces of vata, pitta, and kapha combine to form a constitutional ratio that makes us who we are. In Ayurveda this combination, known as *prakruti,* is the genetic code that remains with each of us throughout our lifetime. We may implement lifestyle, dietary, and environmental changes to live in better balance with our prakruti, but we cannot fundamentally alter our true nature. Doing so is tantamount to flowing against the current of a river and ultimately leads to struggle, disharmony, and unnecessary energy expenditures. It is for this reason that Ayurveda teaches us to understand and embrace ourselves as we truly are, not as we believe we *should* be. True happiness and harmony is achieved through acceptance—both of the uncontrollable force of nature and of ourselves as a product of that force. The Buddha himself received Ayurvedic care and massage and dedicated his life to the understanding and acceptance of truth. As he wrote, "Accept the world as it is, not as it should be."

Ayurveda treats the individual; the instrument of this individualized approach is the doshas. Although there is an infinite number of potential combinations of the doshic forces, Ayurveda classifies individuals into three major body types: the monotypes of vata, pitta, and kapha. The key to living in balance with our own Ayurvedic constitution is to achieve doshic harmony. This does not mean that we should strive for equal proportions of each dosha in our makeup. Rather, we encourage doshic harmony by understanding the inherent ratio of the doshas within our nature and keeping those in balance. In other words, an individual who is mostly kapha in nature will stay mostly kapha through his lifetime. But in pursuing doshic harmony he will learn to avoid certain habits and routines that may inflame his kaphic tendencies. Although it may take a bit more work, a person with one significantly predominant dosha has the same ability to achieve doshic balance as someone with equal proportions of all three doshas.

While considering the body types it is important to keep in mind the main factors that influence our doshic makeup. In the same way that we inherit certain physical attributes from our parents, we acquire a certain percentage of our parents' doshic tendencies. Our constitutional makeup is also influenced by the environmental factors that surround us at birth, including climatic, cultural, and seasonal influences. Being born in a hot, tropical country in the middle of summer, for example, will tend to raise the proportion of pitta in an individual's constitution.

The cultural priorities of the society we live in can also have an impact on our dosha. Our present Western society is a high-vata culture that encourages mental stimulation, communication, and hypermobility. As a result, many people living in the West suffer from vata-related disturbances such as anxiety, information overload, hypertension, insomnia, attention deficient disorder, and chronic fatigue. Even individuals with very little vata in their constitution will often suffer from a vata imbalance due to the hyperactivity of our current society. A vast majority of our work as healers today revolves around understanding and reducing the vata dosha.

A final point to consider before we delve into describing the three main body types is the deep connection between the body and mind inherent within Ayurveda. Each of us has a unique mental nature, or *manas prakruti,* that generally correlates with our physical constitution. An imbalance within our physical body directly impacts the quality of our mental nature, resulting in negative tendencies that differ for each dosha. Sometimes the mental state of a person can provide a powerful clue about his or her predominant dosha. When out of balance, vata individuals tend to experience anxiety and fear while pitta individuals will react with anger and frustration. Easygoing and stable kaphas tend to experience negative emotions in the form of sorrow and depression. Those people who learn to live in balance with their dosha are more readily able to experience positive emotions, such as happiness, peace, and equilibrium.

One of the distinguishing factors of the healing approach of Ayurveda is its attention to the direct causal relationship between the body and mind. Everything that affects the body—including nutrients, breath, exercise, lifestyle, and massage—has a direct impact on the mind. This is the underlying premise of Ayurvedic psychology, which offers an all-natural holistic approach to coping with modern-day anxieties and the quest for inner peace. In performing Thai Yoga Massage according to the principles of Ayurveda, we are thus providing a restorative tonic for both the body and mind.

The first step of integrating Ayurveda into one's life is to become familiar with the three main constitutions of vata, pitta, and kapha. Once you have an idea of your predominant dosha you can start making the necessary lifestyle changes to achieve optimal health and balance. The Ayurvedic constitutional test on pages 195 to 197 will help you ascertain your predominant dosha, and can be used to determine the constitution of your bodywork recipients as well. The constitutional assessment becomes an individualized map that directs the postures, the pressure, and the pace to be incorporated into each person's Thai Yoga Therapy session.

Consider these descriptions of the three doshic monotypes.

Vata Types

Vata individuals have a predominance of the air element, which is manifested in the body as a thin, light frame and a wiry structure. These individuals have long, angular features and thin, coarse hair that is often kinky. Vata skin is usually dry and dark, and these types are most likely to complain of being cold, even in the warmer seasons. They tend to have small, sunken, dark eyes, which are usually dark brown or dull gray in color. They will have small mouths with thin lips, irregular teeth, and receding gums.

Vata types tend to have erratic appetites and irregular digestion that is easily disturbed. Due to the lack of water in their constitution they may experience dryness in the body in the form of constipation and scanty urination. Vata women often have irregular menstrual cycles with acute premenstrual pain and emotional mood swings.

Vatas are creative, artistic people with imaginative ideas that can change direction as often as the wind. They are open and tolerant of others, but due to their sensitive natures they can retreat when anxious or emotionally insecure. Vata people tend to be hyperactive and usually have multiple projects going at one time, which they may have trouble finishing. They often have restless minds; they may speak quickly and suffer from insomnia.

Pitta Types

Pitta persons are governed by the element of fire, which is reflected in their fiery, passionate temperaments. They are hot in nature with a robust circulation that leads to ruddy coloring and warm extremities. They tend to have a medium-sized build and moderate muscle tone. Pitta skin is fair, warm, reddish, and soft. They will burn easily in the sun and have many freckles and moles, with a tendency toward rashes or acne.

Pitta people have average-sized, piercing eyes that tend to be light in color: blue, gray, hazel, green, or yellowish. They tend to have soft, thin, light-colored or reddish hair that may turn gray or bald early. They will be prone to inflammation of muscles and tissues, especially in the shoulders and middle back, where they tend to accumulate stress. Pitta types have a robust, healthy appetite and will become irritable if they skip a meal. They have the best digestion of all three types, with soft, loose bowel movements and frequent urination. Pitta women tend to have regular menstrual cycles with heavy bleeding and premenstrual irritability or anger.

Pitta people tend to be intelligent, powerful, and clear, with a focused mind that makes it easy for them to succeed. They are light but moderately good sleepers and are the type most often to complain of being overheated. Pitta people can be aggressive and competitive in nature, which sometimes causes them to be workaholics and overly

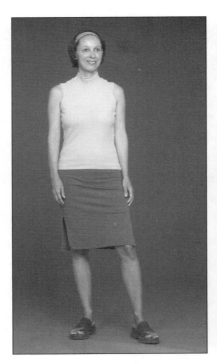

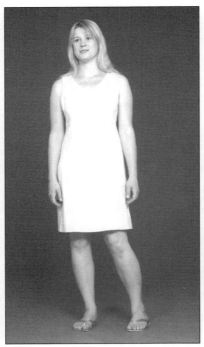

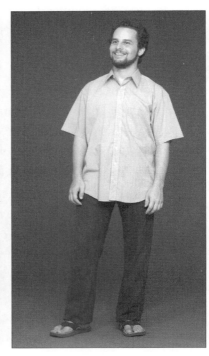

Vata people tend to be thin and narrow, with delicate features and prominent bones.

Pitta people tend to have medium frames, easily inflamed skin, and fiery or light-colored hair and eyes.

Kapha people tend to have large frames with well-developed muscles, soft skin, and wavy hair.

ambitious. If they are not careful, pitta types can light the candle at both ends and suffer from burnout. They are intense people and, when provoked, can become hotheaded and easily angered.

Kapha Types

Individuals of a kapha nature have a predominance of the water element, which is reflected in their full, soft features and moist skin. They tend to have a stocky build, a large frame, and a well-developed chest and will have a tendency to be overweight. Kaphas have thick, soft, oily hair that is often wavy and plentiful. Their eyes are usually large and attractive, blue or light brown in color, with long, thick lashes. They tend to have large, round faces with full lips and big white teeth.

Kapha skin is thick, oily, and cool to the touch. These individuals will have a steady appetite with slow but regular bowel movements and minimal urination. Kapha women tend to have regular cycles with little pain and a minimum of premenstrual depression.

In personality, kapha types are easygoing, fun loving, and patient. They speak and move slowly and have a grounded disposition that is not easily shaken. Their calm and reliable nature makes them ideal managers and caretakers. Kapha types are heavy sleepers, but sometimes they like sleep too much! When out of balance they can be stagnant, sluggish, or overly sentimental, and may find change difficult.

BALANCING OPPOSITES: THE TWENTY ATTRIBUTES

The great Ayurvedic physician Charaka found that everything around us can be defined by a basic set of qualities, or attributes. He grouped these attributes into ten pairs of opposites that reflect the dualistic nature of all existence. The twenty attributes, as described by Charaka, are as follows.

cold/hot	soft/hard
heavy/light	smooth/rough
wet/dry	dull/sharp
static/mobile	gross/subtle
dense/flowing	cloudy/clear

According to Charaka, for every quality there is an opposite quality, and harmony is achieved by balancing these oppositions. This theory of the opposites is at the foundation of Ayurveda and exists within many other Asian healing systems, most noticeably the yin and yang dynamic of traditional Chinese medicine. The principle that *opposites heal each other* is at the basis of all Ayurvedic therapies, including medicinal herbs,

SELECT ATTRIBUTES AS THEY RELATE TO THE DOSHAS

 VATA

Cold	Extreme sensitivity to cold, wind, and dry weather. Cold extremities, such as the hands, feet, and nose.
Dry	Dry skin, hair, and lips. Tendency toward constipation due to dryness in the large intestine. Cracked and hoarse voice.
Light	Physically underdeveloped muscles and body frame. Light-headed, creative thinker. Underweight. Light sleeper.
Swift	Fast to act and react. Quick to change directions, like the wind.
Mobile (irregular)	Rapid walker, taking small steps. Quick thinker and talker. Able to juggle multiple things at once. Sometimes scattered. Variable moods and faith. Restless eyes, hands, feet.
Rough	Cracked and course skin, nails, hair, and teeth. Joints often pop or crack.

 PITTA

Hot (irritable)	Intolerant of heat and direct sunlight. Strong appetite and digestion. Warm hands and skin. Red hair and rosy complexion. Can be hot-headed, fiery, or impatient.
Slightly oily	Moist hands and skin, tendency toward acne. Soft hair.
Light	Medium to light body frame and weight. Piercing eyes.
Liquid	Moist hands; soft and loose joints and muscles. Abundance of perspiration, urine, and thirst. Loose, liquid stools.
Mobile (intense)	Intense minds, like the flame of a fire. Motivated.
Sharp	Focused mind with a sharp memory. Sharp or angular features with pointed nose. Sharp appetite; unable to skip meals.
Soft, smooth	Soft and well-lubricated skin, lips, hair, and joints. Tendency toward strong body odors.

SELECT ATTRIBUTES AS THEY RELATE TO THE DOSHAS (CONT.)

 KAPHA

Cool	Intolerant of cold, damp environments. Tendency toward colds, congestion.
Wet, oily	Oily skin and hair. Well-lubricated joints.
Heavy	Well-developed muscle and body frame; tendency to be overweight. Heavy bones. Deep, heavy, pleasant voice.
Dense	Thick hair, nails, and skin. Slow moving and thinking.
Static, stable	Calm, content, stable personality—"like a rock" or "down-to-earth." Aversion to change. Tendency toward inertia, excessive stillness, or sleep.

diet, gems, mantras, color therapy, and the Ayurvedic cleansing treatment of *pancha karma*. In each of these therapies, excessive qualities are first identified and then substances or actions are applied to counter these qualities. As a basic example, coldness is treated by warmth, dryness by moisture, and lightness by heaviness.

A second important Ayurvedic tenet is *like increases like*. As Charaka writes, "The like is the cause of the increase of all things at all times and the unlike the cause of their decrease; everything that we experience can either increase or decrease similar qualities within our being." For example, a positive state of health can be increased by activities of a similar nature, such as proper rest, yoga, meditation, and wholesome nutrition. On the other hand, factors such as negative thinking, stress, and poor diet will detract from one's overall state of health.

In this book the Ayurvedic principles of *opposites heal each other* and *like increases like* are applied to the practice of bodywork. With an understanding of our recipient's predominant dosha, we can apply the appropriate touch techniques and atmosphere to counterbalance his or her predominant constitution or doshic imbalance. When customized to the unique body type of each individual, the particular massage approach, pacing, and pressure become powerful healing instruments.

As we become familiar with the qualities of each doshic type, the twenty attributes can be observed in those around us. Dryness, for example, is a strong vata attribute that is revealed through dry skin, cracked nails, or dry hair. The opposite attribute of wetness, on the other hand, is found in kapha individuals in the form of oily hair, soft skin, and excessive mucus. By becoming aware of these tendencies, bodywork practitioners are in a better position to identify and address any existing imbalances within the bodies of their clients.

In the table on pages 18 and 19 we have summarized the key attributes that relate to each dosha, with a description of how they are expressed in the body. While the doshas may share attributes among themselves, it is the combination of various qualities that makes each dosha unique. Please note that not all twenty attributes are mentioned in this table, as we have chosen to concentrate on those that relate specifically to bodywork.

SEVEN DOSHIC TYPES

While our application of Thai Yoga Massage styles and moves will focus on the needs of the three main doshic types just discussed, when you combine doshas there are indeed seven types, and it is useful to have some understanding of all of these.

The first group is the monotypes, which we have just discussed. A monotype exists when one dosha is clearly predominant, resulting in individuals with pure vata, pitta, or kapha constitutions. An individual who exhibits a close balance of two doshas is considered a duotype; the three duotypes are vata-pitta, pitta-kapha, and vata-kapha, with the order of the doshas switched according to which is predominant.

A final tridoshic type occurs when an individual has an equal ratio of vata, pitta, and kapha. This occurs very rarely. Most people have two predominant doshas present in their constitution and are therefore considered duotypes.

The general approach to healing in Ayurveda varies according to each of the seven main doshic types. In integrating Ayurveda and Thai Yoga Massage, the best approach when working on an individual with a mono-doshic type involves applying techniques and treatments with qualities opposing those of the predominant dosha. For example, in line with the Ayurvedic rule that opposites heal each other, a pure vata type would be balanced by the application of a warm, slow, and steady Thai Yoga Massage approach. For duotypes, those in whom two doshas are clearly present, the most effective treatment method is to calm the dosha most out of balance. If you are working on a vata-pitta person who is experiencing insomnia and anxiety, for example, you would take a vata-reducing approach to your sessions.

Another scenario that sometimes arises it that the doshas in a duotype individual are equally matched in their predominance. In this case the most effective approach is to increase the third (or least prevalent) dosha. For instance, vata-kapha types are likely to experience coldness or weak digestion due to the lack of fire, or the pitta dosha, in their constitution. These individuals benefit from a Thai Yoga Therapy approach that

HEALING APPROACHES FOR THE SEVEN MAIN DOSHIC TYPES

DOSHIC TYPE	HEALING APPROACH
Vata	Vata-reducing
Pitta	Pitta-reducing
Kapha	Kapha-reducing
Vata-pitta	Kapha-increasing
Pitta-kapha	Vata-increasing
Vata-kapha	Pitta-increasing
Vata-pitta-kapha	Treat specific symptoms and attributes

stimulates pitta through a heating massage, warming aromatherapy or essential oil application, and asanas that stimulate the digestive fire, increase circulation, and heat the body.

In the final tridoshic body type, which you will encounter only rarely, a practitioner would apply techniques that alleviate specific symptoms and imbalances. If, for example, a recipient has an equal ratio of vata, pitta, and kapha but complains of excessive phlegm, the practitioner would apply kapha-reducing techniques to relieve congestion. This is an advanced approach that requires further training in Ayurveda for correct implementation.

THE NATURAL CYCLES OF THE DOSHAS

According to Ayurveda, one of the best methods for achieving doshic balance is following the cycles given us by Mother Nature. Each dosha reaches a high point and a low point during a particular season, time of the day, and period of life. Nature already provides us with the appropriate resources so that we may achieve balance within these cycles. For example, cooling fruits and vegetables, such as watermelon and cucumber, arrive in the middle of the hot summer seasons, and grounding root vegetables, such as yams and potatoes, are ready to harvest during the chilly, windy beginnings of winter. Unfortunately, due to the vast options available to the modern-day consumer, many of us have lost touch with these natural cycles of agriculture. We can now eat berries and melon in the winter and any variety of root vegetable in the summer. When taken on a regular basis, such seasonally inappropriate choices of nourishment send mixed messages to the body and result in inefficiency and imbalance. By educating ourselves and others on the seasonal and daily cycles of the doshas, we can minimize the adverse affects of such consumption. The wisdom of Mother Earth's cycles offers a commonsense approach that is an easy and effective way of integrating Ayurveda into our everyday lives.

Let's consider the seasons and times that can be associated with each dosha.

The season in which vata is most aggravated is the cool, dry, windy season of fall and early winter, and so vata people are particularly sensitive to imbalance during these months. Vata people should take special care during this season to follow a diet, lifestyle, and bodywork approach that is vata-reducing. Frequent massages are recommended for all individuals during this season, particularly for vatas. The time of the day associated with vata is early morning until the sun rises and late afternoon until the sun sets. These are both periods of lightness and activity, when the mind is alert and mobile. If possible, vata individuals should schedule massage during these high-vata periods of the day.

Pitta is most prominent in the late spring and hot summer months, when the temperatures rise and the sun is longest in the sky. Pitta individuals should avoid excessive exposure to the sun during this season and integrate plenty of cooling bodywork as a counterbalance. An evening stroll under the cooling full moon is a good way of reducing pitta in the hot summer season. Pitta types should take special care during high noon and midnight, the pitta time of day when the body is engaged in digestion. A cooling massage during either of these times will provide an effective method of maintaining doshic balance.

THE NATURAL CYCLES OF THE DOSHAS*

	HIGH VATA	HIGH PITTA	HIGH KAPHA
Season	Fall, early winter	Late spring, summer	Late winter, spring
Time of day	Dawn, dusk 3 AM–7 AM 3 PM–7 PM	Midday, midnight 11 AM–3 PM 11 PM–3 AM	Early morning, evening 7 AM–11 AM 7 PM–11 PM

*These are the periods when individuals should take special care to live in balance with their constitution. The ideal time for receiving bodywork is when a person's dosha is at its highest.

During the winter season the temperature drops, clouds accumulate, and precipitation falls in the form of rain and snow. The accumulation of kapha during the winter season begins to defrost in early spring, causing congestion and colds. Winter and early spring are the seasons when kapha individuals need to be most vigilant, following a kapha-reducing diet and breaking up stagnation through exercise and dynamic bodywork. The times of day associated with kapha is midmorning and early evening, when the body feels the most heavy and lethargic. Although sleepy kapha types may avoid physical activity in the morning, this is actually the ideal time for them to receive Thai Yoga Massage!

This chapter has introduced you to the most fundamental aspects of the ancient Indian Ayurvedic system of healing. Much like a work of art, the body is a composition of varied materials existing on different layers. We began by considering the gross material of the five great elements and reflected on the more subtle qualities of the twenty opposites. We then saw how these qualities combine in the body to create the three main Ayurvedic body types. Now that you have gained a comprehensive knowledge of these basics, you are far along the path of understanding how Ayurveda might integrate into Thai Yoga Massage. In the next chapter you will be given the tools to customize your massage according to the Ayurvedic body type of each client.

Customizing a Massage According to Ayurvedic Principles

Once you have determined a recipient's main Ayurvedic dosha, you are ready to design your Thai Yoga Massage according to that client's individual needs. The first key to integrating Ayurveda into a Thai Yoga Massage practice are the three main massage approaches that correspond to each doshic type. Those are the focus of this chapter.

The everyday practices of Ayurveda are deeply rooted in profound concepts of Vedic philosophy. This is especially apparent in the classification of the massage approaches for each dosha.

According to Vedic philosophy, there are three forces of nature within the universe that are present within all matter and are responsible for all creation. As we discussed in chapter 1, these three subtle qualities, or gunas, are known in Sanskrit as sattva, rajas, and tamas. Sattva, generally understood to be the most subtle of the three, is defined as harmony, light, virtue, and intelligence. Rajas is a vital active force that relates to activity, movement, change, and excitability. Our present-day society, characterized by constant movement and activity, is ruled by rajas. The final guna of tamas is considered to be the most gross or material of the three and is associated with heaviness, darkness, and inertia.

Within the practice of Thai Yoga Therapy, the main massage techniques are defined in relationship to these three forces of nature. While one's doshic body type remains the same throughout his or her life, the gunas that determine a person's mental nature are

THE THREE GUNAS

Sattva		The quality of harmony, virtue, or being (sat). It is said to be light and luminous in nature. It is the principle of intelligence.
Rajas		The quality of distraction, turbulence, and activity. It is said to be mobile and motivated. It is the principle of energy.
Tamas		The quality of dullness, darkness, and inertia. It is said to be heavy, veiling, or obstructing. It is the principle of materiality.

transitory. So, regardless of body type, each person has the same ability to evolve and cultivate the sattvic guna in their life. This, in fact, is the underlying aim of Ayurveda and Thai Yoga Therapy—to raise the sattvic nature in ourselves and those around us. As we help ourselves and our clients to achieve doshic balance, we create openings for greater harmony, light, and peace.

MASSAGE APPROACHES AND THE GUNAS

The key to understanding the appropriate guna, or energetic force, to apply to a given doshic body type lies in the fundamentals of Ayurvedic pulse diagnosis.

In the Ayurvedic pulse-diagnosis system, the rhythm of energy flow for each dosha is likened to distinctive qualities of a specific animal. The vata pulse is quick like a snake and slithers around, creating a weak, erratic pulse that is hard to identify. The pitta pulse is strong and rapid like a frog and tends to bound with force and rigor, making it the easiest to recognize. The kapha pulse tends to be slow and graceful like a swan, with profound vibrations that are often hidden deep beneath the thick layers of the kapha skin.

The best way to remember the appropriate palpatory approach for each dosha is to keep a visual image of the animal analogies in mind, along with the Ayurvedic rule of thumb that opposites heal each other. The fast, slithering vata snake is balanced out by a slow, steady pace with the least amount of pressure and long pauses—a sattvic approach. The robust and intense pitta frog requires a steady pace with moderate pressure and pauses—a rajasic approach. And finally, the slow and graceful kapha swan benefits from a faster pace with strong pressure and short pauses—a tamasic approach.

Sattvic Touch

The harmonizing quality of the sattvic approach is most suitable for vata types, who tend to be sensitive in nature and can be overwhelmed by too much stimulation or heavy pressure. The sattvic massage approach is characterized by a light, gentle touch that is done at a slow and easy pace. Of the three approaches, this one involves the least amount of pressure; it is most suited to vata individuals, who tend to be more sensitive to pain and have more delicate bone structures. Although a long, gentle hold may be appropriate in some instances to ground vatas, it should never cause them excessive strain or discomfort. It may be tempting to twist your thin, flexible vata client into a series of challenging postures, but this will actually do her more harm than good. A slow, even pace with frequent repetitions is more appropriate.

The mild, harmonizing sattvic approach balances out vata's tendency toward erratic energy flow, anxiety, stress, and nervous disorders. A safe, pleasant, and nourishing environment can be created with the use of serene music, candles, and a generous amount of plush pillows and blankets. As vata individuals tend to chill easily, make sure that the massage room is at a warm, comfortable temperature.

The best time to massage a vata person is at dawn or dusk, when vata tends to be the highest and most prone to imbalance. In Thai Yoga Massage, the use of therapeutic oils can cause a slippery grip and leave stains on clothing, mats, and pillows. However, it is possible to integrate the use of oil at the end of a massage by applying small amounts to the hands, feet, face, areas of strain, or specific marma points that can be easily accessed without undressing. Use a base oil that corresponds to one's dosha, adding a few drops of essential oil as appropriate for aromatherapy. Sesame oil is a favorite in all forms of Ayurvedic treatment and is especially good for vata types because of its warming, heavy, and pacifying qualities. Warming, earthy aromas such as cinnamon, patchouli, or sandalwood can help to ground vata individuals.

Rajasic Touch

As the rajas guna is a force of activity, it follows that the rajasic approach to massage involves more energy and movement than the sattvic approach. This massage approach is most appropriate for pitta individuals, who require a moderately active massage to release built-up energy and aggression. While pitta types also need to be cooled and calmed, the slow and sedating sattvic approach will leave them feeling frustrated and wanting more. As a middle way, the rajasic touch uses firm pressure with a steady and flowing pace that calms and restores pitta individuals.

Because pitta types may be easily aggravated by excessive heat, the use of force should be monitored and counterbalanced, with a brief pause as an interlude between the more stimulating postures. In general, avoid long holds in the postures, as this can be heating. The aim should be to work through tensions rather than to break up resistance.

MASSAGE APPROACH FOR EACH BODY TYPE

  VATA

Sattvic approach	Gentle massage; light, mild, gentle, balancing, and harmonizing. Less pressure; massage with care and sensitivity.
Best time for massage	Dusk and dawn (high vata time)
Holds	Gentle, long holds with easy repetitions
Oils	Sesame oil to calm and balance the body
Essential oils or incense	Grounding or warming aromas such as almond, frankincense, cinnamon, basil, camphor, ginger, musk, myrrh, nutmeg, patchouli, sandalwood, wintergreen

  PITTA

Rajasic approach	Moderate massage; penetrating and cooling; probing movements. Apply firmness and consistency, but never force.
Best time for massage	High noon or midnight (high pitta time)
Holds	Moderate; avoid long holds, which tend to be heating
Oils	Almond, olive, coconut, brahmi (gotu kola), and sunflower
Essential oils or incense	Cooling, diffusive, and sweet scents such as sandalwood, gardenia, lavender, lotus, jasmine, rose, vetiverian. Apply to third eye and temples to cool the head.

  KAPHA

Tamasic approach	Strong massage; heavy, deep, fast, opening, and clearing. Use force, intensity, and determination.
Best time for massage	Late morning or late evening (high kapha time)
Holds	Long dynamic holds, with some repetition as needed
Oils	Avoid most oils or apply small amounts of light oils, such as safflower or sunflower oil.
Essential oils or incense	Stimulating and invigorating scents such as bergamot, camphor, cloves, eucalyptus, ginger, mint, musk, myrrh, peppermint

Steady, probing movements can be used to expel toxins, aid digestion, alleviate muscular tension, and relieve knots. During energy-line work, take care not to over-thumb or over-palm your pitta recipients, as these techniques increase circulation and have a heating effect on the body. Also, excessive rubbing may irritate sensitive pitta skin, which is prone to rashes and inflammation.

The best time for a pitta person to receive a massage is at high noon or midnight, when the sun's effect is most powerful and needs to be relieved. If using oils for localized application, pittas benefit from light or cooling oils such as sunflower, olive, or coconut. Sweet and calming floral scents such as rose and lavender, or the cooling scent of sandalwood, are also recommended.

Tamasic Touch

The quality of tamas is characterized by heaviness and solidity. The tamasic massage approach involves the deepest and most rigorous touch techniques. This massage approach is suitable for kaphas, whose thick, oily skin requires the most stimulation.

Kapha individuals benefit from a strong, heavy, and forceful bodywork approach that breaks up stagnation and accumulation. The pacing for this massage is the fastest of all three approaches and involves intensity and determination on the part of the practitioner. The aim is to open up the body and circulate stagnant energy on the physical, mental, and emotional levels. Kaphas may love to receive a soft and soothing massage, but following the Ayurvedic rule of thumb that opposites heal each other, such an approach would only plunge them into a deeper state of slumber. Of the three primary doshic types, kaphas can handle long holds with some exertion—so you can save your most dynamic Thai Yoga Massage moves for them! Of course, this may be difficult if you are a small vata person working on a heavy-framed kapha individual. In these cases remember to follow common sense and never sacrifice your own comfort or safety.

The use of well-paced repetitive movements, such as rotations and stretches, can help to open up the body and get things moving. The best time for massaging your kapha clients is in the late morning or late evening, when this force is strongest in the body.

Finally, because kaphas already tend to have oily skin and hair, it is best to avoid most oils or to apply small amounts of light oils, such as safflower or sunflower. Stimulating, energizing scents that open the nasal passages, such as eucalyptus or mint, benefit kapha individuals and can be applied to the chest and nose in cases of heavy congestion.

AREAS OF ACCUMULATION

Within the Ayurvedic system, each dosha is associated with particular parts of the body where its forces tend to accumulate. In order to deepen the therapeutic quality of a Thai Yoga Massage session, it helps to know the areas of the body at which each doshic type tends to accumulate tension and metabolic waste.

Each type has a main site of accumulation that is located in the gastrointestinal tract, and it is here where undigested food mass, or *ama,* tends to build up. When ama is allowed to accumulate over an extended period of time, it can overflow and relocate from the gastrointestinal tract into the weakest areas of the body. Disease occurs when ama collects in such weak pockets of the body and becomes irritated or "angered."

The key to preventing ama buildup is strengthening *agni,* or the body's internal digestive fire. The level of agni determines how well an individual absorbs food and discharges the waste products of the body. When agni is sufficient there is no toxic buildup in the body and mind. When agni is insufficient, however, we suffer from improper digestion, dullness, heaviness, stagnation, and cloudiness. Hence, the state of agni is essential to the health of the body within the Ayurvedic system.

Maintaining healthy functioning of the digestive fire is comparable to keeping one's home furnace running smoothly. Regular maintenance checkups and the use of appropriate fuels ensures a safe fire and the prevention of residue buildup in the furnace. Similarly, the digestive fire of agni is maintained by regular health checkups and a nutritional, lifestyle, and bodywork program that corresponds to one's predominant dosha. As a preventive treatment, Thai Yoga Therapy helps to increase agni, reduce the buildup of ama, and draw the bodily toxins back to the sites of accumulation. In cases of high ama buildup a more extensive Ayurvedic detoxification known as *pancha karma* is necessary; this requires the expertise of a qualified Ayurvedic physician.

The fact that the principal site of accumulation for each dosha is located within the digestive system reflects the importance of proper nutrition and digestion within Ayurveda. The main site of accumulation for vata people is the large intestine or colon. Vitiated vata often manifests in the large intestine in the form of constipation, excessive gas, irregular bowel movements, or lower back pain. Other vata-related areas of the body to be aware of while performing a massage include the spine, back muscles, thighs, kidneys, bones, and the hollow cavities of the body, such as the ears and the pelvic bowl. Very often you will find that vata recipients carry tension or have disturbances in these areas, so you may want to draw your healing awareness to these areas during a massage session.

For a pitta person, the main site of accumulation is the small intestines, where the digestive juices act as a fire for the system. Excessively high pitta often expresses

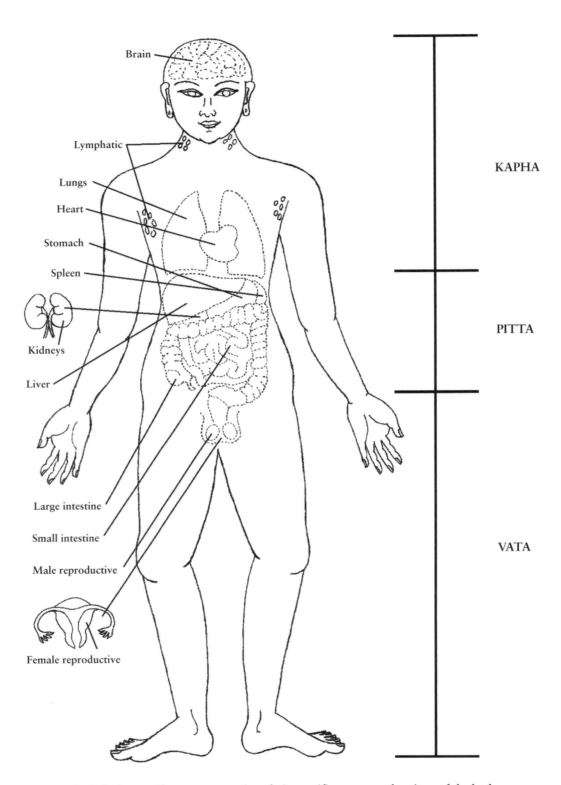

Brain

Lymphatic

Lungs

Heart

Stomach

Spleen

Kidneys

Liver

Large intestine

Small intestine

Male reproductive

Female reproductive

KAPHA

PITTA

VATA

Each dosha manifests more prominently in specific organs and regions of the body.

THE DOSHAS AND ORGANS / REGIONS OF THE BODY

 Vata's site of accumulation: Colon
Other key vata areas: Spine, back muscles, thighs, kidneys, bones, hollow cavities of the body, such as the pelvic cavity and ears

 Pitta's site of accumulation: Small intestines
Other key pitta areas: Mid-abdomen, upper hips, liver, spleen, eyes

 Kapha's site of accumulation: Stomach
Other key kapha areas: Chest, lungs, sinuses, nose, throat, head, joints, pancreas, lymph nodes, synovial fluid

itself in the form of irritable bowel syndrome, acid indigestion, heartburn, ulcers, or diarrhea. The subsidiary sites for pitta, and thus other sites to keep in mind during a massage session, include the mid-abdomen, upper hips, liver, spleen, and eyes.

The main site of accumulation for a kapha recipient is the stomach. Vitiated kapha often expresses itself in the form of weak digestion, low appetite, and nausea. Excessive kapha also accumulates in the lungs and respiratory system in the form of mucus and congestion. Other areas of the body related to kapha include the sinuses, nose, throat, head, joints, pancreas, lymph nodes, and synovial fluid.

According to Ayurveda, all disease begins with ama, identifiable in the Sanskrit word for disease—*amaya*. It is easiest to flush away ama when it is still located in the respective site of accumulation: the large intestine for vata, the small intestines for pitta, and the stomach for kapha. Ayurveda uses diet, herbs, yoga asanas, steam therapy, and massage to draw the disease from the body and return it to the original site of accumulation. Once the ama has returned to the gastrointestinal tract, customized massage sessions aid to flush the toxins from the site of accumulation and out of the body.

Whether one requires a sattvic, rajasic, or tamasic touch, the practitioner should never apply a massage approach in a formulaic way that overlooks the unique limitations or desires of the client. If a person requests a massage approach that does not Ayurvedically match his or her body type, never force the issue. In these cases it is best to offer a nonintrusive explanation as to why another approach might be suitable, but then leave the decision up to the client. People who are living in a state of imbalance often crave a food or lifestyle that is the opposite of what they need; this applies to their desired massage approach as well. In order for the wisdom of Ayurveda to be truly beneficial, an individual must actively choose his or her own path to self-awareness and healing.

It is important to use common sense when applying any massage approach to avoid injuring yourself or your recipient. Never force a massage approach on a client who specifically requests another style. Appropriate modifications should always be made in cases in which injuries or medical conditions may be aggravated by any of the massage approaches. The elderly and people with fibromyalgia, cancer, AIDS, osteoporosis, or any disease causing frailty should always receive the light and gentle massage of the sattvic approach. (Individuals with a medical condition should always first seek the advice of a physician before receiving a massage.) When beginning a massage session it is recommended to start with a sattvic touch to relax the body before applying a more rigorous approach, even if your client requires a rajasic or tamasic touch.

AN INNER JOURNEY THROUGH THE KOSHA BODIES

While working on the level of the gunas we are providing an individual approach that touches on all of the five yogic *kosha* bodies. The koshas, extensions of the physical body, have five forms or sheaths. The first is the physical body, the *annamaya kosha*. The second, the energy body or *pranamaya kosha*, is a layer of life force just above the skin. *Manomaya kosha*, the third layer, is the mental body, where thoughts and doubts are experienced. The fourth is the intellectual body, the *vijnanamaya kosha*, which provides one's identity and sense of self. The fifth is the *anandamaya kosha*, the blissful body that allows one to connect with the metaphysical.

Obstruction to the free flow of energy results in an insufficient supply of prana. This can lead to mental, physical, and spiritual imbalances within the kosha bodies, which may manifest in the form of disease, discomfort, or emotional problems.

The five *koshas*, or "bodies," constitute a map of therapeutic healing starting at the gross physical body and moving toward the more subtle layers, ultimately leading to our core self: the embodied soul (see table on page 33). This inner journey is representative of the experiences a person undergoes in a lifetime, in a period of reflection, or even during a session of Thai Yoga Massage. Through working with the body we are able to integrate the energetic fields of the five bodies, expanding our energy out to reach the bliss sheath.

During a Thai Yoga Therapy session we begin by working on the physical body, or *annamaya kosha*, enabling the recipient's muscles, joints, skin, and bones to relax and align. Physical touch, massage approach, and Thai Yoga Massage postures all catered to the recipient's doshic type bring awareness to the body, wake up the senses, and channel energy to various parts of the body. The recipient's breath is deepened, thus enabling a greater awareness of the breathing process and an expansion into the vital essence body of *pranamaya kosha*. As we will discuss, this expansion is aided by an

THE KOSHA BODIES AND THAI YOGA THERAPY

KOSHA BODY	HEALING GOAL	HOW THAI YOGA THERAPY HELPS ACHIEVE THIS GOAL
Annamaya kosha (physical body)	To honor one's physical self	Greater awareness of the physical body Proper body mechanics and alignment Nutrition, exercise, and lifestyle suited to one's body type
Pranamaya kosha (vital essence body)	To increase, cultivate, and balance one's pranic self	Synchronization of breath and body in movement Energetic massage that engages the five vayus Deep rhythmic breathing and awareness of breath Pranayama home exercises
Manomaya kosha (mental body)	Inner peace and equilibrium of mind	Customizing the massage according to one's dosha promotes balance and calmness in the mind Deep relaxation, letting go of emotions and the chattering mind
Vijnanamaya kosha (intellectual body)	Understanding oneself and universal truth	As the first three koshas become more integrated, one slips into a deeper state of relaxation This allows for deeper insights about oneself and the universe
Anandamaya kosha (blissful body)	Meeting of universal and individual mind	Integration of all five kosha bodies brings about a union of body and mind. Connection to one's radiant core, growing sense of wholeness, unconditional love, acceptance and inner peace

Ayurvedic understanding of the five forms of prana (the *vayus*), sen-line work, marma point therapy, and the appropriate breathing techniques for each dosha.

As the body enters into a deeper state of relaxation and awareness, the *manomaya kosha*, or mental body, becomes calm and still. The ups and downs of the chattering mind are neutralized, allowing for the internal stillness of the mind to emerge, much like the lake bottom comes into view when the waves disappear. The mind is further stabilized with the integration of a customized wellness therapy program that includes a home yoga practice, breathing and meditation techniques, nutritional attention, and supportive lifestyle changes.

With the synchronization of the body, breath, and mind the intuitive knowledge of the intellectual body, or *vijnanamaya kosha*, unfolds. During this stage of the massage the recipient may have deeper insights about herself and the nature of the universe as a whole. Such awareness leads to a greater sense of freedom and an understanding of the true compassionate self and the interconnectedness of all beings.

Feeling relaxed in the body and mind, the recipient falls into a deep state of peace and tranquility experienced through the *anandamaya kosha,* the blissful body.

By integrating the knowledge of the kosha bodies into our massage work, we also evolve as practitioners—moving from a physical approach to a more holistic energetic level of healing. The most essential method for understanding energetic healing in Ayurveda involves the concept of the vayus, or five subtle movements within the body. We will now turn our discussion to the vayus, the final tool enabling us to customize a therapeutic approach based on Ayurvedic principles.

THE VAYUS

The ancient Vedic text *Chandogya Upandishad* refered to subtle energies that flow through the body as "gatekeepers of the celestial world." These mysterious healing energies are known as the *vayus;* they control the direction and circulation of life force throughout the body. *Vayu,* Sanskrit for "wind," can be imagined as a continuous flow of energy that moves like a current in five principal directions: upward, downward, outward, inward, and centrally. The movement of the five vayus controls and animates the entire body, enabling us to breathe, move, communicate, receive nutrients, and expel wastes. Obstructions or incorrect flow of the vayus can lead to emotional and physical imbalance and, in many cases, disease.

Working with the subtle energies of the vayus is one of the main purposes of Ayurvedic massage. Much like learning a new language, communicating with the vayus requires awareness, sensitivity, and repeated practice. By mastering these energies we can encourage the directional flow of prana to address the specific doshic needs of our clients, significantly increasing the healing benefit of our practice.

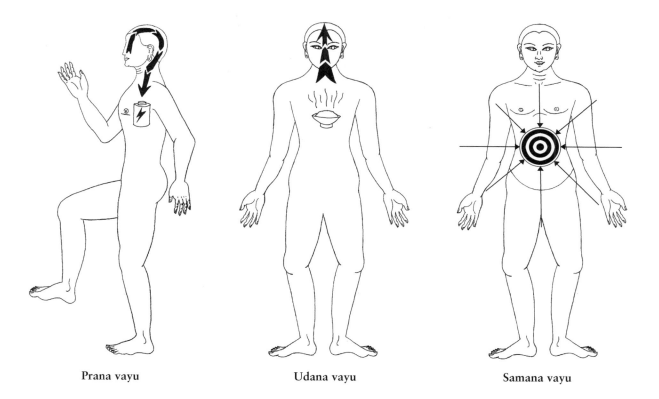

Prana vayu

Udana vayu

Samana vayu

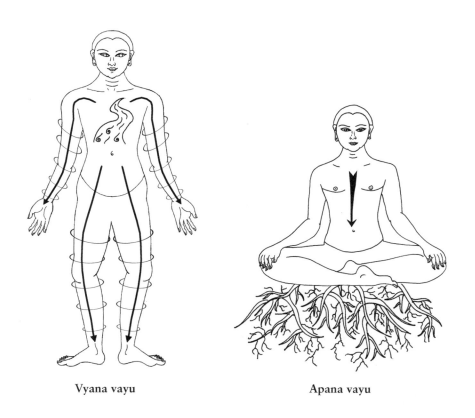

Vyana vayu

Apana vayu

The first direction of the inner wind is known as *prana vayu*. It is present in an individual's cranial cavity and moves downward and inward into the head, throat, heart, and lungs. The prana vayu should not be confused with the general prana, or life force, of the body; it is a subtype of prana. Prana vayu is the most controlling of the five vayus and is responsible for determining a person's overall health. It governs inhalation and is associated with the recharging of our internal vital energy. Prana vayu is responsible for sensation, feelings, perception, and the circulation of thoughts. It is generally considered to be neutral in temperature. The primary movement of prana vayu is inward.

The second direction of wind flowing in the body is *udana vayu*. It is centered in the diaphragm and moves upward through the lungs, throat, senses, and brain, all the way up to the crown of the head. Udana vayu governs exhalation and is responsible for coughing, sneezing, speaking, and memory. The upward flow of energy has a heating effect. The primary movement of udana vayu is upward, creating a lifting sensation in the body.

Samana vayu, the third direction of wind in the body, is directly connected to the digestive system. It is related to the contraction of energy at the navel and small intestines that creates hunger, stimulates the secretion of digestive enzymes, and governs proper absorption. Samana vayu can be imagined as a bellows used to maintain a steady and continuous burning of the body's digestive fire, or agni. As a result of its function in temperature control, this vayu is linked with lowering excess heat. It has a cooling effect on the body. This vayu is associated with a centralization of energy and linear movement into the belly button.

The opposite of the contracting movement of samana is the expanding movement of *vyana vayu*. Vyana is centered at the heart and pumps the internal wind to the body's extremities, circulating blood, nutrients, and oxygen throughout the body. Vyana vayu governs reflex actions and coordination within the muscular and skeletal systems. This vayu is responsible for circulation and therefore, like udana vayu, has a heating effect on the body. The primary movement of vyana vayu is circular and expansive.

The final direction of the five vayus is the downward movement of *apana*. This vayu is related to the process of elimination that expels all the metabolic waste materials

The Five Vayus

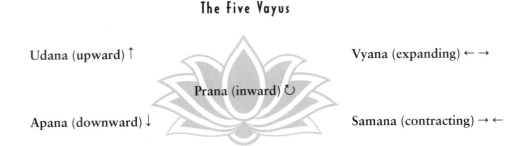

Udana (upward) ↑   Vyana (expanding) ← →

Prana (inward) ↺

Apana (downward) ↓   Samana (contracting) → ←

down and out of the body. Apana vayu is present in the colon, the rectum, and the urinary tract. It governs defecation, urination, flatulence, and menstruation and childbirth. Apana vayu is associated with downward movement; by releasing excess heat it has a cooling effect on the body.

The five vayus can be easily remembered as consisting of one primary force, or prana vayu, and two pairs of opposites, as illustrated in the diagram on page 36.

THAI YOGA MASSAGE AND THE FIVE VAYUS

Knowledge of the vayus is an effective key to the interface between Ayurveda and bodywork practices such as Thai Yoga Massage. By tapping in to the vayus the practitioner is able to work at a deeper, more energetic level and direct the flow of energy through the recipient's body. Pranic energy can be channeled according to the doshic needs of the client, fostering deep healing, recovery, and restoration.

Vamadeva (Dr. David Frawley), author and founder of the American Vedic Institute and a pioneer on this subject, has provided extensive research on the movement of the vayus in his book *Yoga for Your Type: An Ayurvedic Approach to Your Asana Practice*. Inspired by Dr. Frawley's research, we have developed a system for identifying and sensing the vayus in Thai Yoga Massage. Each Thai Yoga Massage pose activates one or several of the vayus within the recipient's body; the vayus associated with each pose are clearly outlined in the massage form in part 3 so that the practitioner may begin to connect with the energetic potentials of the vayus. After some practice an intuitive understanding of the vayus will emerge and this initial process of analysis and thinking can be shed.

Below we will explore the characteristics of each vayu and the Thai Yoga Massage movements that naturally increase or decrease the flow of each vayu. Pay special attention to the heating, cooling, or neutral quality of each vayu, as this can be particularly useful for balancing an individual's doshic constitution.

Prana Vayu ↻   Best for: Vata

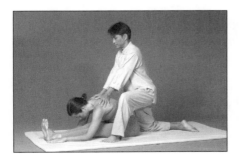
Forward bend

Characteristics of prana vayu: Energizing— inward movement, increasing vital energy; neutral temperature

Site: Head, moving down and in toward the throat, heart, lungs, and diaphragm

Prana vayu is increased by forward bends, inwardly directed postures, pranayama breathing exercises.

The movements most closely associated with activating prana vayu are forward bends, marma point pressure, and pranayama, or yogic breathing exercises, such as *anuloma viloma* (alternate nostril breathing). Forward-bending postures encourage the recipient to surrender and turn his attention inward. Postures that engage prana vayu tend to have a neutralizing effect on body temperature, thereby relieving excessive heat or cold. By closing off to outside distractions and excessive stimulation, the recipient experiences an inner recharging of his or her innermost vital essence. For this reason, prana vayu is most beneficial to vata types, who typically exhaust much of their energy by responding to external disturbances.

When working on vata clients, imagine that you are channeling the prana vayu to the center of the body to recharge the pranic battery. By regulating the prana vayu, we help our clients to conserve their energy reserves and avoid depleting their energy levels. This is especially important for vatas, who tend to have bursts of energy that become quickly frittered away, leaving them emotionally and physically exhausted.

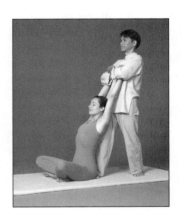

Udana stretch

Udana Vayu ↑   Best for: Kapha

Characteristics of udana vayu: Ascending movement; heating

Site: Diaphragm, moving up through the lungs and throat and up to the crown of the head

Udana vayu is increased by the dynamic movement of raising hands or legs, and by inverted postures.

Any movement that draws the recipient's attention to the cranial region and area just above the head stimulates the upward flow of udana vayu. This includes poses with the extremities extended above the body, such as overhead arm stretches, leg raises, or inversions. The rush of blood to the upper extremities, head, face, and sensory organs tends to have a heating effect on the body. A good example of a Thai Yoga Massage posture that encourages upward movement is Udana Stretch. This upward surge of energy awakens the mind and senses, making it ideal for mobilizing stagnant kapha types. When working on kapha clients, the use of dynamic and aerobic movements can help to counter this body type's slow and inert pace, opening the body and removing blockages. The breathing technique of *kapalabhati,* which involves a rapid succession of forcible expulsions through a pumping of the abdomen, also engages udana vayu.

Vyana Vayu ← →

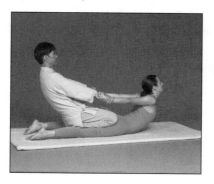

Cobra pose

Best for: Vata and kapha

Characteristics of vyana vayu: Expanding—outward movement; heating

Site: Heart, moving throughout the body to all extremities; promotes arterial and venous circulation

Vyana vayu is increased by backbends, extending poses, spinal twists, traction, rotations, palming, and thumbing.

The outward flow of vyana vayu mobilizes the blood to circulate oxygen and nutrients to all of the body's extremities. Postures that generally increase vyana vayu include backbends, extensions, spinal twists, tractions, and rotations. For example, Cobra pose provides an upper backbend that stimulates the heart and increases arterial and venous circulation. Vyana vayu is also stimulated by the Thai Yoga Massage techniques of palming and thumbing, which increase circulation and waste removal within the bodily tissues. Working along the sen energy lines is particularly good for promoting an outward flow of blood from the heart, which washes away lactic acid buildup.

In general, all circular motions can be associated with vyana vayu, including the rhythmic rocking technique of whirlpool rock, which stimulates vyana vayu in the practitioner and receiver. (The rhythmic rocking techniques will be covered in chapter 5.) This vayu is also stimulated during the Thai Yoga Massage technique of blood stop on the arms and legs, which creates a rush of blood through the body. The outward and expanding distribution of blood has a heating effect on the body and for this reason is suitable for balancing the cooler doshas of vata and kapha.

Samana Vayu → ←

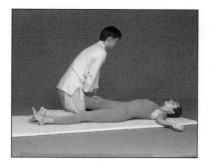

Demi Diamond

Best for: Pitta and vata

Characteristics of samana vayu: Contracting—consolidated, centralized, or introverted movement of digestion to balance agni (digestive fire); heating

Site: Small intestines, moving around the navel and out to the large intestines

Samana vayu is increased by sitting poses, bound postures, and mild spinal twists that tone the liver, spleen, and stomach.

Samana vayu is a contracting and centralized flow of energy that occurs around the navel in preparation for digestion and absorption. Samana vayu governs the secretion of liver enzymes, the proper functioning of the gall bladder, and the regulation of appetite. Postures that can be associated with activating this vayu include bound postures, mild spinal twists, and all sitting poses that promote stability such as the Demi Lotus and Demi Diamond. These movements help to activate samana vayu by consolidating the body's energy and channeling it to the digestive fire of agni, which is responsible for maintaining proper metabolic balance.

The palming of organ reflex points during the abdominal massage is particularly good for promoting samana vayu and proper digestion. For example, the Thai Yoga Massage posture Demi Diamond enables an efficient channeling of digestive energy that has a cooling effect on the body. For this reason, postures that activate samana vayu are particularly suitable for pitta types.

Apana Vayu ↓   Best for: Vata and pitta

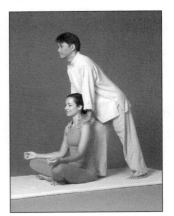

Palming Shoulders

Characteristics of apana vayu: Descending movement; cooling

Site: Colon, pelvic cavity, urinary tract, and reproductive organs, moving downward and outward

Apana is increased by comfortable sitting postures that stabilize the legs, lying postures, squatting, and downward movement of the abdomen.

Apana vayu is the downward and outward movement of the body that is responsible for eliminating waste products that exist on both the physical and mental levels. Sitting, squatting, and lying down postures promote relaxation and allow for waste to surface and be expelled from the body. Apana energy is activated while we sleep, which on the mental level is evident by the release of anxiety and negative thoughts in our dreams. On a physical level, apana vayu is present in the need to evacuate the bladder and bowels shortly after waking. Palming Shoulders stimulates a downward movement that follows the natural flow of gravity downward and out. Apana vayu is also associated with postures that release excess "wind," or vata, in the body, such as Demi Lotus, a variation of the Wind-Relieving yoga asana. The well-loved Thai technique of toe cracking is another example of how excess wind is expelled from the body.

THE VAYUS AND THE DOSHAS

A well-balanced Thai Yoga Massage session or yoga practice will engage all five vayus: providing energization (prana), expansion (vyana), contraction (samana), upward movement (udana), and downward movement (apana). However, we can cater a session by channeling those vayus that are most appropriate for each constitutional type. As you integrate this knowledge into your practice, remember that the vayus are subtle energies that require a sensitive and meditative approach to practice. Mindful awareness and directed intention can increase the healing benefits of each vayu discussed.

The most important vayu to connect with for our light, airy, vata types is the grounding, downward movement of apana vayu. Vatas also tend to have erratic and weak energy levels and for that reason they benefit from the inwardly restorative effect of prana vayu. While working on a vata client, the one vayu you should avoid is the upward movement of udana, as this tends to "space out" and deplete vata. Samana and vyana are also beneficial for vata as the former stimulates digestion and the latter circulation, both areas of weakness for vata people.

Pitta recipients generally benefit from a cooling flow of samana vayu that pulls excess heat from the extremities inward toward the abdomen. Apana vayu is also good for pittas as it drains excess heat from the head and upper body and moves it to the lower extremities. Pittas should avoid postures that overly activate the heating vayus of udana and vyana.

Kapha practice should primarily focus on increasing the upward movement of udana to bring lightness, energy, and stimulation to the body. The most effective way to activate udana is through inverted postures and poses in which the recipient's arms and legs are extended over her head. Postures that activate circulation through vyana vayu also benefit kapha. Kaphas should avoid forward bends, which contract the chest, and too many sitting and lying poses, which activate the stabilizing vayus of apana and samana.

VAYU APPROACH SUMMARY

DOSHA	ENGAGE	AVOID
Vata	Apana, prana	Udana
Pitta	Samana, apana	Udana, vyana
Kapha	Udana, vyana	Samana, apana

Perhaps the most effective method of connecting with the five vayus is to experience these subtle energies firsthand within your own body. The following meditation, based on the work of Dr. David Frawley, is a good means for exploring the vayus.

To practice this meditation, sit in a comfortable position, close your eyes, and listen to these words spoken by another person or by your own recorded voice.

Take a deep inhalation. Imagine the prana entering your nose and traveling inward, toward your cranial cavity and head. The movement of prana vayu continues downward and inward toward your throat, lungs, diaphragm, and heart. Prana vayu governs inhalation. Take a few deep breaths.

On your next inhalation, feel the prana moving from the diaphragm upward into the lungs, bronchi, throat, sinus cavity, and all the way up to the crown of your head. This is udana vayu; it is responsible for governing exhalation. With each exhalation notice a lifting sensation expanding upward through the body.

Inhale deeply, allowing the breath to expand into your belly. Feel the prana moving into your abdomen. As you continue to breathe into the abdomen, draw your attention to the linear movement around the navel, stomach, and small intestines. This is samana vayu. As you exhale, notice that the abdomen naturally contracts, releasing excess heat in the digestive region. With each inhale draw new energy to the region, enabling the secretion of enzymes and digestive juices for proper digestion and absorption.

Now draw your attention to your heart. On your next exhalation imagine the prana traveling from the heart and expanding outward to all the extremities of the body, extending into each and every finger and toe. This is vyana vayu. Continue to breathe deeply and more rapidly than normal. Feel a heating sensation as your breath circulates oxygen to all regions of the body.

Take a deep inhalation. As you exhale feel a downward sensation throughout the body, as if you are being pulled down with the natural force of gravity. This is apana vayu; it governs the body's waste removal and reproductive system. On your next inhale draw your attention to your pelvic cavity, colon, urinary tract, rectum, and reproductive organs. Exhale and follow the breath downward and out, tracking the path of elimination for all food, water, and negative thinking.

In this chapter we have considered several techniques for customizing Thai Yoga Massage according to the Ayurvedic needs of our clients. We began with the three main massage approaches that can be applied to counterbalance the predominant constitution of our recipients. We also discussed the areas of accumulation in the body for each dosha. Finally, we introduced the concept of the kosha bodies and the vayus, which unveil the energetic potential within Thai Yoga Therapy.

In the following chapter, we conclude our discussion of massage approach by reflecting on energy-line work and marma point pressure for each dosha. Ideally, each of these techniques should be integrated into a massage practice in an intuitive way that does not follow a formulaic pattern. The Japanese samurai swordsmen learn their skills through a series of detailed exercises studied carefully, one at a time. After many years of training, they retire to the mountains to meditate until they have forgotten what they have learned. When the swordsmen return, they have so naturally integrated the knowledge into their style that they are directed by intuition rather than thought.

Just like the swordsmen, we too need to begin by learning the precise techniques of customizing a massage according to Ayurvedic principles. Once we have integrated this knowledge into our style, we can abandon the specific details and let intuition guide us.

Energy Points and Pathways

The *gopi chant* is an ancient Indian instrument that consists of a stick, a cone, and a string. This simple musical device makes an enchanting and natural sound that often sets the rhythm and background for singing, chanting, or reciting poems. The gopi chant is a one-stringed instrument that is so approachable that, with some practice and discipline, just about anyone can play it.

A similar statement can be made about the art of sen energy-line work, which is also based on intuition and natural rhythm. According to the yoga philosophy upon which Thai Yoga Therapy is based, there are 72,000 energy lines running through our bodies. Of these lines, ten are of key importance to Thai massage. These lines, known as the *sip sen,* connect the marmas, or pressure points, throughout the body. Massaging the sen promotes the free flow of prana through these important energy hubs.

SEN ENERGY LINES

The Ayurvedic foundation of Thai folk medicine can be recognized by comparing details of the Thai sen energy-line system and the Indian *nadi* energy-line system. The three principal lines for each system follow identical pathways; in addition, the nomenclature for both systems is remarkably similar. For example, Sen Sumana (from Thailand) and Sushumna nadi (from India) both refer to virtually the same energy line.

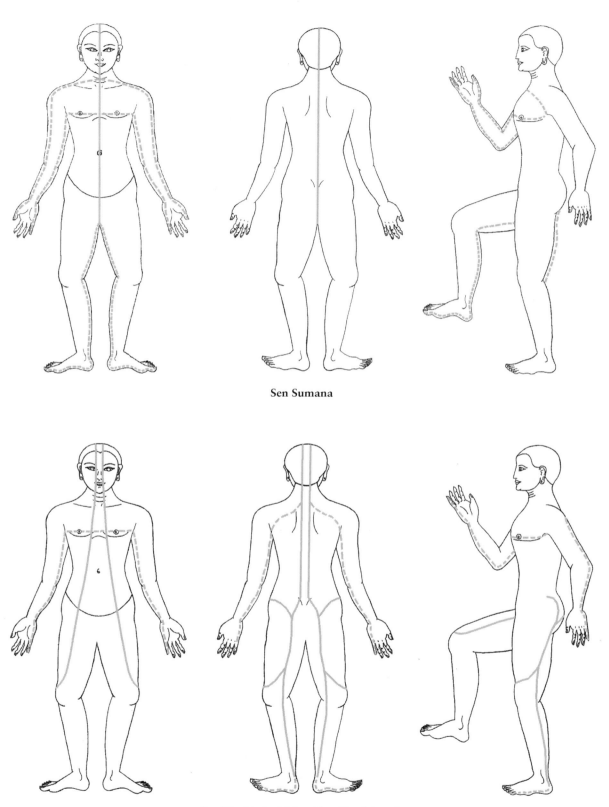

Sen Sumana

**Sen Pingkhala (right side of body) and
Sen Ittha (left side of body)**

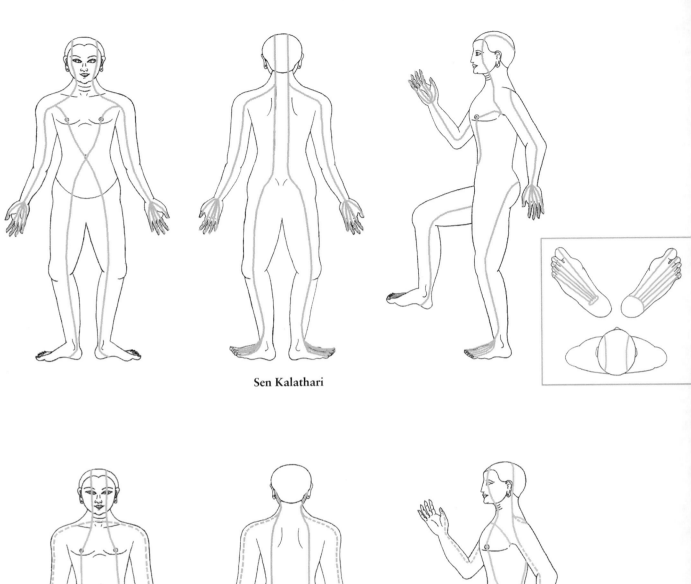

Sen Kalathari

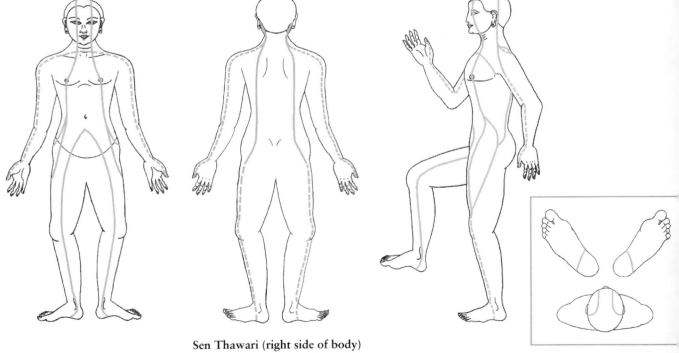

Sen Thawari (right side of body)
and Sen Sahatsarangsi (left side of body)

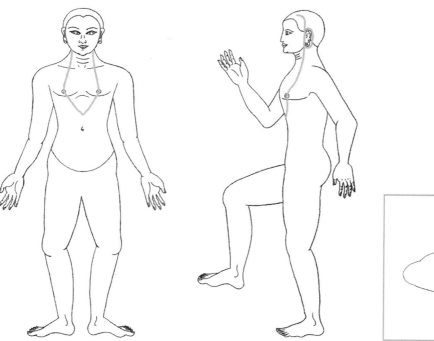
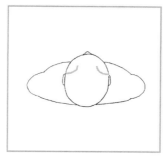

Sen Ulangka (right side of body)
and Sen Lawusang (left side of body)

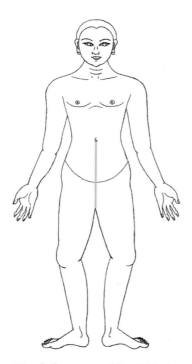

Sen Nanthakrawat and Sen Khitchanna
(These lines run nearly parallel, with Sen Nanthakrawat
following the reproductive pathway and Sen Khitchanna
following the elimination system.)

This line runs from the coccyx through the seven chakras to the crown of the head. The two names are spelled differently but have a similar pronunciation and meaning. The same is true for the right line of the body, which is referred to as Sen Pingkhala in Thailand and Pingala nadi in India. The left line of the body is known as Sen Ittha in Thailand and Ida nadi in India.

Through assisted yoga postures and therapeutic touch techniques that tone the musculature of the body, Thai Yoga Massage balances the entire network of sen energy lines, releasing tension and revitalizing the body. By opening the body in this way, energy flows more easily; this enhanced energy flow helps alleviate common problematic conditions such as lower back pain, arthritis, headaches, digestive difficulties, menstrual problems, and stress-related conditions.

In Thailand the teaching of sen energy lines differs according to geographic and regional location. Some of the most respected schools teach multiple interpretations of the same energy-line system; even in the same village one might find two masters teaching different locations and healing properties for the same sen lines. On the surface this may seem contradictory and confusing, but the healing results of these master masseurs cannot be denied. We have observed these healers enter into a deep meditative state that transcends the limitations of any physical landmark or location—in effect, they feel the location of the lines through an intuitive touch, loving-kindness, and a devotion to healing. There are many interpretations of the sen energy-line locations, but with the correct intention and spirit any devoted practitioner will be able to practice and master this system.

The best method for working on the sen-line system is to embody a relaxed and playful energy that will encourage you to open up to your intuition. In Thai Yoga Massage we work the energy lines through muscle palpation, assisted yoga asanas, and stretches. Every individual has a unique body, and for that reason the exact pathways and locations of the lines run differently for each person. It is therefore impossible to apply a predetermined energy-line map to all of our clients. The knowledge of the sen energy-line system provides us with a strong theoretical base to begin our energy-line work. Yet, if we get stuck on following these details too rigidly, we risk staying in our heads and ignoring the true needs of our clients. Instead of working from the intellect, our approach to energy-line work must be centered from the heart.

As you place your hands on your client in preparation for the sen energy-line work, notice the quality of your thoughts. At first you may find yourself thinking about the precise location of the lines as illustrated in this book, or perhaps as you learned them during a recent workshop. Over time, as your confidence builds, you should become less dependent on these supports and instead allow intuition to direct your work. Rather than referring to external resources that teach the general location of the lines, you will find yourself turning inward to listen to the energetic composition of each client. When approached in this way, sen energy-line work generates a deep state of relaxation and promotes centeredness and well-being for both the client and the practitioner.

Similar to the vayus discussed in the previous chapter, each doshic type has a unique flow of energy throughout the body that requires an individualized approach to sen-line work. The flow of energy in a vata person, which tends to be quick and erratic, requires a steady, slow approach to palpation; kapha people, on the other hand, benefit from an invigorating approach that breaks up stagnation and allows energy to flow more freely through the sen lines and marmas. By gaining an understanding of these subtle nuances, Thai Yoga Massage practitioners can listen well with their hands and adjust the sen work according to the Ayurvedic constitution of their client.

The analogy of the three pulses to certain animals, introduced in chapter 3, provides useful imagery as we personalize the palpatory approach for our recipients. For vatas, palpation of the muscles and sen energy lines is best performed at a meditative, slow, and regular rhythm that helps to calm and equalize vatas' erratic energy flow. Slow, moderate pressure that gradually increases circulation and promotes deep breathing is most effective. The strong and fiery energy flow of pittas makes these individuals vulnerable to excessive circulation and overheating. Pittas therefore benefit from a cooling approach that does not overstimulate blood circulation or irritate sensitive pitta skin. However, if the pace is too slow, a pitta person may become frustrated or bored. A moderate pace with light pressure is most beneficial for these individuals. Kapha recipients will tend to have a more slow, sluggish energy flow, and for that reason are best suited to an energizing pace that breaks up physical and mental stagnation. A strong and firm pressure will enable the kaphic "river of ice" to thaw, releasing toxins that may facilitate a burst of new energy. Of all the doshas, kaphas requires the most rapid pace for sen-line and muscle palpation.

THE MARMAS

Another important element in an Ayurveda and Thai Yoga Massage session is working the pressure-point system of the marmas.

Pressure-point therapy is an ancient healing art practiced in many Asian cultures. Along the sen pathways are concentrated points, energy centers like spiraling whirlpools that can either retain energy or radiate energy outward. In the Indian tradition these energy centers are called *marmas*. Often when we fall sick it is because of energy blockages or imbalances in the marmas. By applying pressure to these points we can help to promote a strong energetic flow throughout the body and thereby alleviate common ailments and relieve pain.

Physically speaking, a marma is an anatomical location in the body where two or more types of tissue, such as muscle and tendon, meet. A marma point can range in size from the diameter of a penny to a small plate—such large proportions makes the science of marma-point therapy more user-friendly than other varieties of pressure-point therapy. In addition to being centers of cellular mass, marma points are hubs for the vital and subtle energies of the body. When these points get obstructed or blocked in some way, there is insufficient flow of prana and energy throughout the body. This can lead to a disruption of our doshic harmony, leaving us vulnerable to fatigue and illness.

According to the classic Ayurvedic text *Susruta Samhita,* there are 107 marmas on the human body. Seven of these major marma centers are situated along Sen Sumana; these seven marma centers are popularly known as the seven major chakras. When massaging any of the marma points, unnecessary tension that hinders the free flow of prana is released. When the centers of distribution in a plumbing system are clogged, water flows more slowly and inconsistently through the pipes, thereby making the overall system inefficient. By working on the marma points we are "unclogging" the blockages and promoting proper circulation through all of the bodily and energetic channels, including the five kosha bodies. Because a Thai Yoga Massage treats the individual on the physical, energetic, emotional, mental, and spiritual levels simultane-ously, the recipient may not only be assisted physically, but she may also enter inner territories to begin addressing fears and deep-seated anxieties that may be hindering her progress in some area of life. When done with mindfulness, marma therapy is a profound healing modality that can help remove blockages and restore a greater sense of physical and mental equilibrium.

As with other classical Indian disciplines, such as yoga, dance, and music, the ancient knowledge of marma point therapy is part of an oral tradition that has been passed on through the generations. The precise details of marma location and therapeutic appli-cation are traditionally recorded on palm leaves, hidden away and shared with only the closest disciples, who themselves will carry the tradition to the next generation. Such secretive roots have led to differences in the practice of marma point therapy from region to region across India. But, although these discrepancies may seem contradic-tory at first, they actually add to the richness and therapeutic strength of the practice. Rather than scientifically memorizing a marma "blueprint" for all individuals, prac-titioners are encouraged to rely on a deeper sense of intuition in order to treat each recipient's body as unique.

Of course, there is a need for memorization when first learning the marma system, but with constant practice and awareness an intuitive understanding emerges. Eventu-ally it is possible to transcend the conditioned and self-limited mind and attune oneself to the vital energy of each recipient. A form of pranic healing emerges in which the practitioner directs his or her own prana to improve the recipient's flow of energy. In this way the practitioner's own pranic practice is just as important, if not moreso, than the exact location and properties of each marma point.

In the ancient Vedic text *Vasishta Samhita*, a work fundamental to our current understanding of marma therapy, it is written that "one should practice concentration by drawing one's prana by the power of attention from each of these marma regions." As Dr. David Frawley states, often the prana of the practitioner is as important or more important than what we give or do for our patients. All healers should therefore strive to develop their own pranic reserves by following the appropriate diet, yogic practice, lifestyle, and pranayama exercises most suited to their Ayurvedic type.

Marmas are most easily stimulated by pressure applied with the thumb, the main pranic channel in the hand. However, for some marma points the index finger, knuckle, heel of the hand, elbows, arms, knees, and feet can be used. As you work on the marmas, visualize each point as an essential transfer station that passes vital energy throughout the region. Encourage the free and peaceful flow of energy through each transfer point. Direct your own breathing to the marma point, inhaling positive healing energy and exhaling negativity and tension. You may also direct your recipient to breathe into a marma point that seems particularly tender or stagnant.

When experiencing marma pressure your client may feel a range of sensations—a delicious sense of release, a stimulation of energy, or a sense of lightness directly following the removal of pressure. There is nothing more satisfying as a practitioner than finding that point in a client that triggers the well-known utterance of "Ahhhh." If your client experiences pain while you are working on a particular marma, there may be a blockage or stagnant energy occurring at this point. In such cases, only work as deeply as your client is comfortable and never cause excessive discomfort.

Sometimes recipients will endure excruciating pain and maintain a serene external composure—all in the name of "no pain no gain." There is a sense in Thailand that if a massage is not painful enough to conjure tears, the therapist might not be fully seasoned. Pain is viewed very differently in the West and is generally not welcomed during a massage, so you should always ask your recipient to notify you of any sharp or uncomfortable sensations. Because pain is subjective, a helpful technique is to ask for your recipient's feedback using an indicator of 1 to 10, with 10 being the maximum intensity. We should always respect the physical needs and cultural expectations (as far as we can know them) of our recipients, and never exceed an intensity level of 5.

The position, healing attributes, and massage application for each marma point are discussed in further detail in part 2.

This book offers an easy and effective path for integrating Ayurveda into a bodywork practice so that you, as the practitioner, may help yourself and others achieve doshic harmony and balance. The process of harmonious living presented here involves two steps: first becoming aware of your own tridoshic nature according to Ayurveda, and then applying this knowledge to help others.

The unfolding of this process is a universal pathway of self-discovery that can strengthen our roles as healing practitioners, but the journey *must* begin with our own bodies. It is only by having a good understanding of our personal Ayurvedic body type and existing imbalances that we can begin to discern the constitutions of others. As we take steps to live in balance with our own true nature, a greater sense of clarity and inner peace arises, awakening new levels of prana and intuitive force.

Much like the process of learning a new language, understanding Ayurveda and applying its principles to inform our Thai Yoga Therapy practice involves viewing the world in a new and integrated way. It is only by immersing oneself in this new way of perceiving that the subtle nuances of Ayurveda are revealed. When Thai Yoga Massage is practiced in partnership with the medicine of the Buddha, a new healing potential emerges.

PART 2

❖

The Physical Elements of Thai Yoga Massage

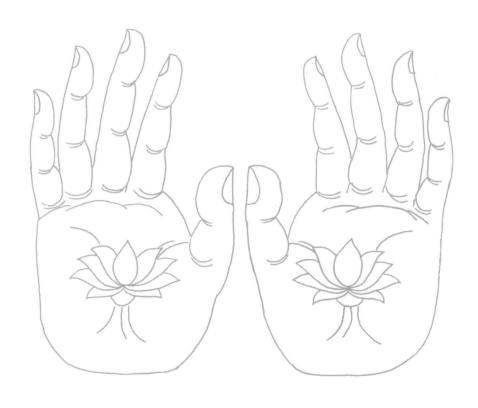

Thai Yoga Massage Stances and Touch Techniques

Now that we have discussed the Ayurvedic foundations of Thai Yoga Therapy, in this next part of the book we will consider the tools and techniques essential to a successful practice of Thai Yoga Massage.

At the Lotus Palm School we incorporate four basic tools into every aspect of a massage: mindful awareness, rhythmic rocking, working stances, and therapeutic touch techniques. Employing these four tools, the Thai Yoga practitioner maintains proper body alignment, fluid body movement, and steady and consistent compression, all the while assessing the physical needs and range of motion of the person receiving the massage.

These four tools remain at the heart of the Thai Yoga Massage practice, whether the person giving the massage is a beginner or is a more advanced practitioner. The meditative rhythm that emerges as the synergistic result of properly applying these tools instills confidence in the recipient, ushering him or her into a deeply restful, healing state.

MINDFUL AWARENESS

Because customizing a massage according to the Ayurvedic needs of a client requires conscious intention on the part of the practitioner, the first and most important element in any Thai Yoga Massage session is the practice of mindful awareness. Mindfulness heightens the sensitivity to touch, encourages good body alignment, and creates a sacred healing space. The more mindful one becomes, the less energy is required in performing a pose. In this flowing dance, Thai Yoga Massage emerges as an effortless art form that benefits both the practitioner and receiver; for the truly mindful Thai Yoga Massage practitioner, every posture becomes a multilayered experience full of subtle nuances that can be freshly perceived with each session.

Because a Thai Yoga Massage session is so deeply physical and involves intertwining arms and legs with the recipient, the practitioner who is not mindful might end up in an awkward posture that could lead to misunderstandings or preventable injuries.

Before beginning a massage the practitioner should take a moment to empty the mind and draw his or her attention to the doshic needs of the recipient. This can be accomplished by simply observing the quality of our thoughts and gently reminding ourselves to return to the present moment. Throughout the massage the mind may wander to contemplate past events—for example, reviewing a recent conversation—or to the future, perhaps thinking about our dinner plans. Yet these distractions take away from our ability to be fully present and listen to our client for signs of physical discomfort, energetic blockages, or emotional release.

Mindfulness is the anchor that draws the practitioner's awareness to the other three basic tools—the rhythmic rocking dance, the working stances, and the touch techniques. (For those familiar with Kam Thye's first book, the following material also appeared in *Thai Yoga Massage*.)

THE RHYTHMIC ROCKING DANCE

Rhythmic rocking dance is the essential movement within Thai Yoga Massage. This technique involves the practitioner swaying his or her body in a rocking motion such that the practitioner's weight creates a natural and even pressure on the recipient's body. With straight arms and a straight spine, the practitioner moves back and forth in a swaying rhythm that resembles the movement of a bamboo reed. The pacing is repetitive but not overly mechanical. The practitioner embodies the smoothness of a cat as it walks, the motion gently rocking the recipient's body, as if cradling a baby to sleep. This calming dance sets the pace for the entire bodywork session.

The movement of the rhythmic rocking dance is like a tai chi movement meditation; you learn how to play with the circular energy of chi and to use the least amount of effort to achieve maximum results. When we hear the word *massage* we usually think of using our hands and thumbs to squeeze muscles. But if you know how to use your whole body in the rhythmic rocking dance when giving a massage, you can conserve energy and avoid becoming exhausted. You can also prevent the development of chronic stress syndromes in the hands, arms, and shoulders.

Instead of using your muscles, the rhythmic rocking dance maximizes your energy by allowing it to circulate down the spine. The energy is then centered within the second chakra—the swadhisthana chakra, the space three fingers below your belly button—and flows into your arms and palms. When you dance this dance successfully you actually borrow energy from the earth. This way, even when you apply a good amount of pressure in the course of a session, you do not feel tired at the end of the massage.

The rhythmic rocking dance is the base for three floor techniques used in working with clients; these techniques are the bamboo (side) rock, the forward rock, and the whirlpool or circular rock. The practitioner applies one of these rocking techniques at a time. The postures in part 3 include recommendations as to which rocking technique is best to use with each posture.

Bamboo Rock (Side Rock)

In the bamboo rock the practitioner kneels, knees spread or pressed together and the tops of the feet on the mat forming a solid base. Tuck the chin in slightly to straighten the spine; the alignment from crown to coccyx should be pure, yet relaxed. Straighten your arms and shift the trunk of the body from side to side, swaying the torso like a bamboo in the wind.

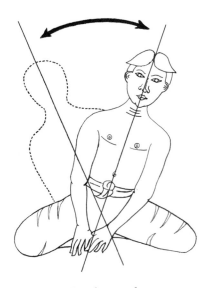

Bamboo rock

Forward Rock

In the forward rock the practitioner begins again by kneeling, knees spread or pressed together and the tops of the feet on the mat forming a solid base. Tuck the chin in slightly, straightening the spine. The alignment from crown to coccyx is straight but relaxed. Maintaining this alignment, rock the torso forward and backward, like a rocking chair.

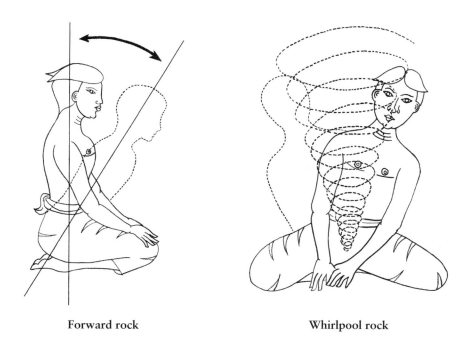

Forward rock   Whirlpool rock

Whirlpool Rock (Circular Rock)

In the whirlpool rock the practitioner begins as above: knees spread or pressed together and the tops of the feet on the mat forming a solid base. Tuck the chin in slightly to straighten the spine; maintain a strong yet relaxed alignment from crown to coccyx. Keeping this alignment, circulate the torso clockwise or counterclockwise in a whirlpool motion, using the coccyx as the axis.

THE WORKING STANCES

Thai Yoga Massage is a beautiful dance that requires continuous movement by the practitioner to provide a relaxed and flowing session for the recipient. It is therefore extremely important that the practitioner uses his body well, moving with effortless, graceful transitions. Ancient lessons regarding fluid movement and the use of proper body mechanics have been extracted from the traditions of tai chi and yoga to create a foundation for the working stances described below.

When holding a working stance within Thai Yoga Massage, consider the tree as inspiration. Imagine your arms and hands are the branches—they are strong, yet yielding. These "branches" are connected to your spine, which is the trunk of the tree, sturdy and erect. The spine transfers your body's weight to your feet, which are the roots of the tree, firmly planted in the earth. By keeping your spine straight and your head up, you are aligning the seven energy centers (the chakras) along the spine. Combining the energy of earth and heaven, like the tree, with the energy of your body, you maintain a strong yet resilient posture that is fluid in every aspect of its movement.

A common mistake for bodywork practitioners is hunching through the back and losing strong spinal alignment through the course of a session. When the body is hunched over in this way, the practitioner is using her shoulders instead of connecting her body to the earth. This position can result in a sore back and fatigue for the practitioner and a less-than-effective massage for the recipient. Always keep the image of the tree present in your body as you practice these stances.

The three rocking techniques of bamboo rock, forward rock, and whirlpool rock can be applied with any of the stances described below. When applying pressure that alternates from side to side, use bamboo rock; for frontward movement or pressure, use forward rock; and for any circular techniques, use whirlpool rock.

Diamond Stance
Kneel on the mat with your knees together, buttocks resting on your heels. The tops of your feet are flat on the mat.

Open Diamond
Kneel on the mat with your knees spread apart and your buttocks resting on your heels. The tops of your feet are flat on the mat.

Kneeling Diamond
Stand up on your knees, your body forming a plane from your knees to the crown of your head. Tuck your tailbone slightly and keep your back erect.

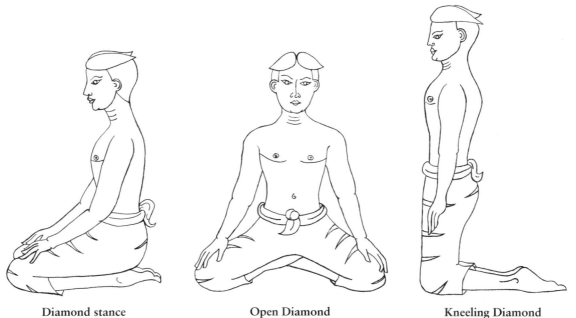

Diamond stance   Open Diamond   Kneeling Diamond

Archer Stance

In a squatting stance, the toes of both feet are tucked under. Place one knee on the ground. Keep your back straight. This is a tricky pose, requiring strength and balance. Practice, practice, practice.

Open Archer Stance

From Archer stance, maintain a straight back and spread your knees apart.

Tai Chi Stance

Stand with feet shoulder-width apart; legs are straight but knees are soft. Step forward a comfortable distance, straightening your back leg and bending your front knee slightly. Do not let your bent knee extend past your toes. The front foot is pointing directly ahead and the back foot is naturally turned outward. Maintain a stable center, with 70 percent of your weight on the front leg and 30 percent on the back leg.

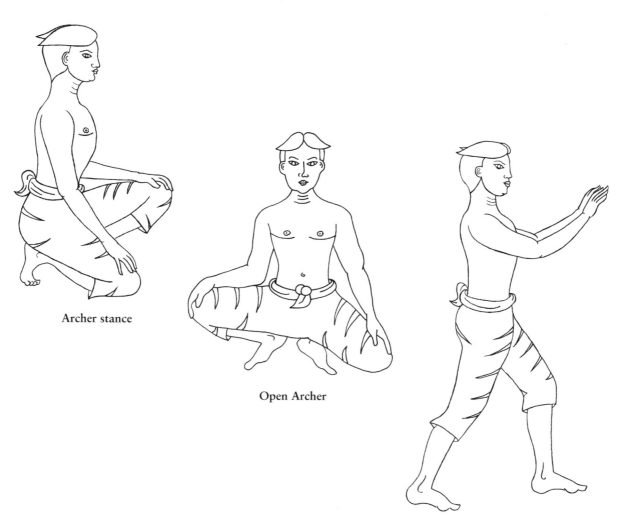

Archer stance

Open Archer

Tai Chi stance

Warrior Stance

From Kneeling Diamond stance, raise up one knee. Keep your arms and back straight. Be careful that the raised knee does not extend beyond the toes. The front heel is grounded. Warrior is the most frequently used stance in a Thai Yoga Massage session.

Open Warrior

From Warrior stance, open your raised knee to the side so that it is at a 90-degree angle to the body. Keep your back straight and your torso facing front.

Horse Riding Stance

Stand upright with your legs a little more than shoulder-width apart and your feet open to the sides. Slowly bend your knees while maintaining a straight back. Do not allow your knees to extend beyond your toes.

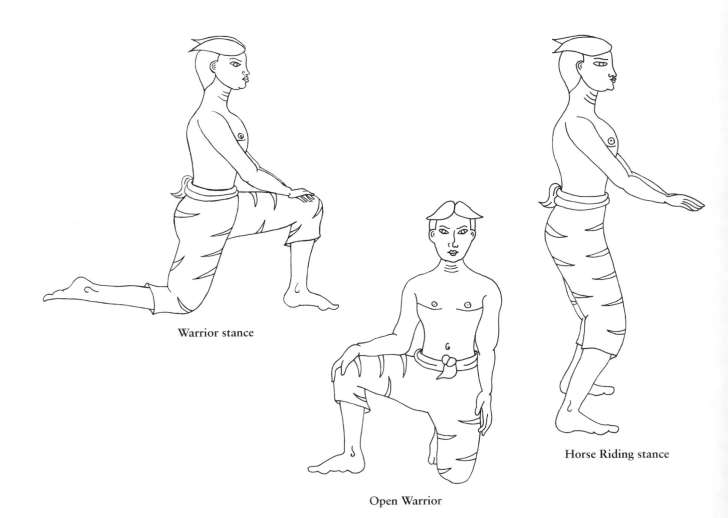

Warrior stance

Open Warrior

Horse Riding stance

Wag the Tail

This transitional movement is often used in Thai Yoga Massage. (In Lotus Palm trainings we refer to the lower leg as the "tail.") From Warrior stance, pivot the back foot inward at a 45-degree angle to the body. To return to Warrior Stance, "wag" your lower leg outward to its original position.

Thai Yoga Massage is a very physical form of therapy—a treatment, which typically takes one to two hours, is often an athletic workout for the practitioner. The key to the practitioner feeling energized, rather than depleted, following a session has to do with the employment of proper body mechanics.

Practitioners frequently overuse the muscles of the hand and the upper shoulder; they also commonly make the mistake of bending the arms, curving the back, and tilting the head downward. While this posture may feel more natural than the working stances described above, it actually disconnects the upper body from the lower body, leading to weakened rapport with the recipient.

In traditional Chinese medicine the three energies of earth, heaven, and body are called the three treasures. These energies are made manifest in our bodies as *ching*, the energy we are born with; *chi*, the energy of life force; and *shen*, the energy of inner heart or spirit. By physically aligning the body in the working stances described here, we allow these three treasures to unite. That unity brings strength to our bodywork session.

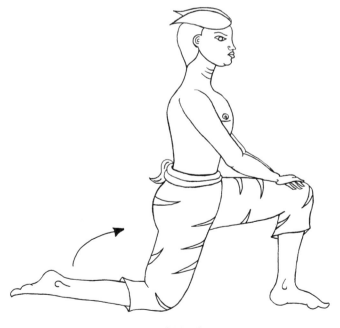

Wag the Tail

TOUCH TECHNIQUES

The manipulations that are most frequently employed in Thai Yoga Massage are the techniques of palming and thumbing. Palming is generally used to open and warm up the body and stimulate the energy lines before beginning the technique of thumbing.

The Thai Yoga Massage series in part 3 is a thumb-saving form that has been specifically designed to use a range of body parts as tools for the massage. Besides the techniques of palming and thumbing, the forearms, elbows, knees, and feet can be used as well.

Palming

In palming, the practitioner uses the area of the palm close to the heel of the hand to compress the energy lines of the recipient's body. You must not use the heel of the hand exclusively, as this could feel like a stick poking into the recipient's body. When palming, cup your hands with your fingers slightly spread, as if you're holding on to a basketball. (Be careful not to overflex your wrist, as this could lead to injuries over time.) Keep your arms and back straight but not rigid; your head is aligned on your spine. From this position, fall in to the recipient's body with your weight, using bamboo rock or forward rock.

Thumbing

Thumbing is a technique that can best be described as thumb chasing thumb. Using his full body weight, the practitioner uses the bamboo or forward rock to press his thumbs into the recipient's body. As with palming, the practitioner keeps arms and spine straight. This sets up a supportive posture for using the thumbs sensibly, an essential element in avoiding overuse injuries as well as providing the most comfort to the recipient.

The correct method for thumbing is to use the pad of the thumb; common mistakes are hyperextending the thumb or pressing the thumbnail into the recipient.

Using Forearms

The forearms are used for smoothing and rolling the muscles in preparation for deep-pressure work on the recipient's body. The practitioner places the forearm on the recipient's body, gradually rocking in with the body's weight as the forearm rolls away from the practitioner. Take care not to use the bony aspect of the forearm, close to the elbow; the ulna bone can be sharp and produce an unpleasant feeling for the recipient.

Using Elbows

Elbows are very effective tools if the recipient requests deep pressure. The elbows are used to apply direct pressure on a specific part of the body. Place the elbow on the recipient's body and, with a relaxed shoulder and upper body, gradually lean in with the full weight of your body. To prevent the elbow from slipping you can hook the

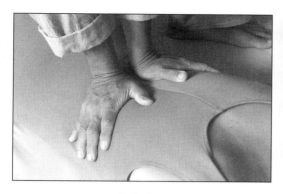

Palming

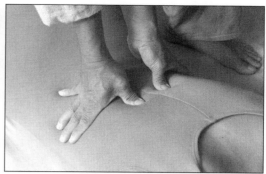

Thumbing

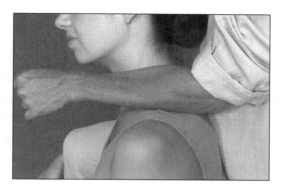

Forearm rolling

thumb and forefinger of the opposite hand around the elbow. Continue using the hand as a guide along the recipient's body.

Using Knees

The knees can produce an even more powerful effect upon the recipient's body than the elbows. The use of the knees demands good balance and agility on the part of the practitioner.

Positioning your hands on the recipient as support, place the knees on the recipient's body. Gradually lean in with your body weight—sparingly, as the appropriate amount of pressure is difficult to judge.

Using Feet

The feet have many nerve endings, enabling them to be as responsive as the hands in giving and receiving information. The feet can be used for applying direct pressure as well as for stabilizing the recipient in postures and stretches. The numerous parts of the foot—the heel, instep, blade of the foot, dorsal, ball of the foot, and toes—can be used in countless ways in the massage. The foot is as versatile as the hand; this should be kept in mind when giving a massage.

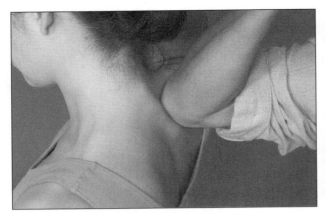
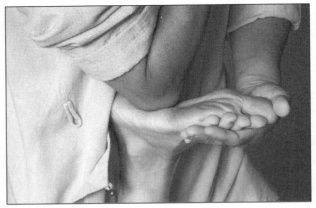

Elbow pressure. The elbow provides an alternative technique for applying deep pressure and is effective in preventing injuries of the hands and wrists due to overuse.

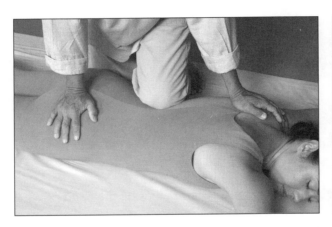
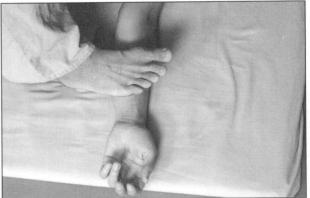

Kneeing   Using the feet for palpation

STAYING CONNECTED

Practicing mindfulness throughout the massage will keep you connected with the recipient and aware of the recipient's response to the firm pressure and deep stretches of Thai Yoga Massage. Our students often ask us how much pressure should be applied during the bodywork session. The best gauge is to start off with a gradual application of your body weight, and then ask the recipient for feedback.

In a Thai Yoga Massage session, the rhythmic rocking dance evens out the energy released in the practitioner's body during palming, thumbing, and forearm or foot massage. Yet, while developing a sense of self-awareness and movement as a practitioner is integral to the successful practice of Thai Yoga Massage, it should not overshadow the importance of being attentive to the recipient. Keep a close rapport with the recipient throughout the session by constantly watching for changes in facial expressions and muscle tension. Oftentimes recipients will not tell you how much pressure is too much. In general, the way the body is feeling is communicated through the face. If the recipient cringes, be sure to reduce your massage pressure or the extent of the stretch.

Here are five points to help you stay focused on the needs of the person to whom you are giving a Thai Yoga Massage.

- Maintain the meditative openness of moment-to-moment awareness.
- Cultivate contact with your recipient by "listening" with your hands and body, keeping regular eye contact, and paying attention to your intuition.
- Respect the recipient's physical, emotional, and sexual boundaries.
- Synchronize your breathing with the pace of the massage and be aware of the recipient's breathing.
- Uphold the tradition of Thai Yoga Massage by basing your practice on mindfulness, loving-kindness, and compassion.

The Thai Yoga Massage techniques and skills introduced in this chapter provide a foundation that will enable you to blossom as your work progresses. By staying in touch with these basics you are ensured a safe, secure, and mindful massage practice. As Kam Thye says in his workshops, "If you follow these basics, you cannot go wrong!"

With our feet firmly grounded in core Thai Yoga Massage techniques, we are ready to branch out and consider the energetic work that occurs when we massage the marma points and sen energy lines.

Working the Sen Lines and Marma Points

According to Ayurveda, there are 107 vital energy points, or marmas, that exist throughout the human body. These points are important hubs of pranic energy that can be stimulated to increase energy flow, remove blockages, or even tap into hidden energy reserves.

The translation of the Sanskrit word *marma* is "secret" or "hidden." Such mysterious undertones to marma theory can be traced to the original application of the science of the marmas within the Indian martial art form known as *kalari payat*. Marma points are broadly classified as either lethal for injuring the enemy or therapeutic for protecting oneself. According to the *kalari payat* tradition, there are twelve marma points that can cause sudden death.

Traditionally, the exact location of the lethal and therapeutic points has been considered a sacred and protected knowledge; as such, it has been passed orally across the generations from teacher to student. In many parts of Kerala in southern India this ancient tradition is still honored, as *kalari payat* masters will only teach the exact location of marma points to their most senior students.

Acquiring in-depth knowledge of the marmas requires many years of hard work and one-on-one study with a reputed master. However, an introductory knowledge of some key marma points provides an insight to the profound therapeutic value of this system.

DOSHAS AND MARMA POINTS

As with the acupuncture points in traditional Chinese medicine, each marma point relates to specific organs or tissues within the body. Marma points are thus identified with one or more of the tridoshas, in correspondence with the sites at which stagnant energy tends to collect for each dosha. (See the discussion of accumulation sites in chapter 3.) For example, when working on kaphas, who tend to accumulate stagnant energy in the lungs, one might stimulate the Talahridaya lung marma point at the center of their feet and palms.

The eighteen marmas selected for the Thai Yoga Massage form taught in this book are considered by most masters to be major points by virtue of their strong therapeutic values. Because of their size and location, these points are also among the easiest to work on within a Thai Yoga Massage format. The exact location of each marma and its therapeutic qualities have been identified following the research of Vamadeva (Dr. David Frawley) and the books of Swami Sada Shiva Tirtha and Ayurvedic medical doctor Hans. H. Rhyner. Seven of the marma points presented here directly correspond to the seven chakras, the vital energy centers aligned along the spinal column. By stimulating these points during a massage session we are effectively releasing a flow of energy throughout the entire chakra system.

The position, healing attributes, and doshic applications of each marma point are detailed in the table on pages 70 and 71. We have also included a drawing of the eighteen marma points used in this massage for ease in locating them.

Marmas are most easily stimulated by pressure applied with the thumb, the main pranic channel in the hand. However, the index finger, knuckle, heel of the hand, elbows, arms, knees, and feet can also be used with many of the marma points. In alignment with the three main massage approaches, the amount of recommended pressure varies according to the doshic needs of your recipient—gentle for vatas, moderate for pittas, and deep for kaphas. For localized marma pressure therapy at the end of the massage, you may wish to apply a small amount of the base oil that corresponds to the recipient's dosha, and add a few drops of essential oil. (For appropriate base oils see the table Massage Approach for Each Body Type on page 27.) Mahanarayan oil is a classic Ayurvedic blend of up to several dozen herbs that is suitable for all three doshas. This therapeutic oil has been used for centuries in India to relieve muscle and joint pain and can now be found in many Ayurvedic supply centers in the West.

All oils should be applied in the direction of hair growth and should be left on the marma point until the recipient's next shower.

Before beginning to apply marma pressure, bring your full awareness to the therapeutic properties and location of the specific marma point you will be working on. Apply gentle pressure with your thumb and gradually pour in with your body weight.

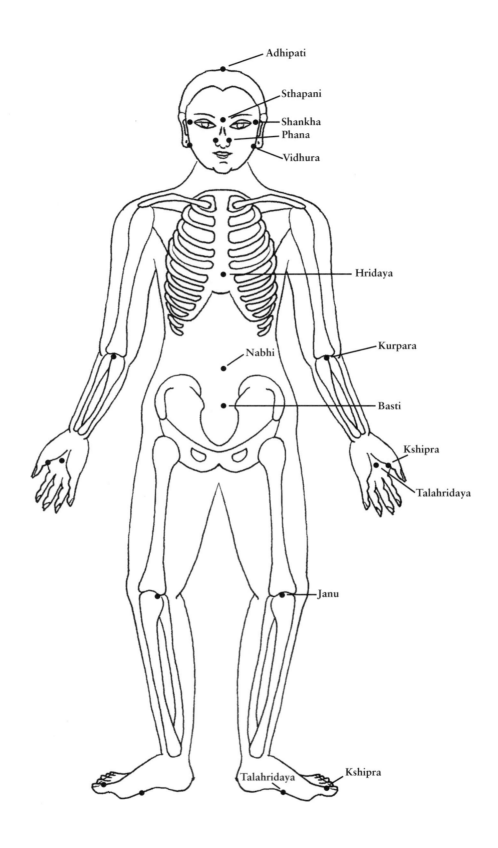

Adhipati

Sthapani

Shankha

Phana

Vidhura

Hridaya

Kurpara

Nabhi

Basti

Kshipra

Talahridaya

Janu

Talahridaya

Kshipra

Key marma points: Front view

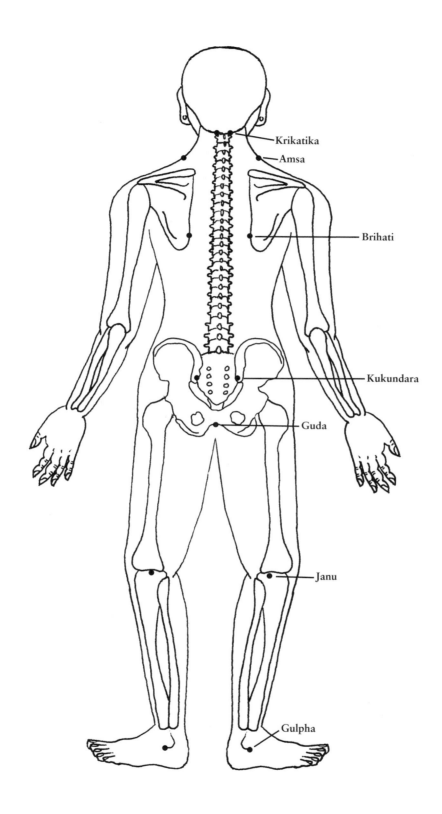

Krikatika

Amsa

Brihati

Kukundara

Guda

Janu

Gulpha

Key marma points: Back view

18 KEY MARMA POINTS

MARMA POINT	LOCATION*	THERAPEUTIC QUALITY	RELATED DOSHAS**
Adhipati marma	Crown of the head, summit of the skull	Controls the seventh chakra (sahasrara, head chakra). Governs the mind and connects to universal energy. Regulates the nervous system, stimulates pineal gland.	Tridoshic
Sthapani marma	Third eye, between the eyebrows	Controls the sixth chakra (ajna, the third eye). Governs the senses; stimulates the pituitary gland.	Tridoshic
Shankha marma	Either side of the forehead, at the hollow point on the temple	Stimulates the colon; relieves tension headaches.	Major vata point
Phana marma	Both sides of nose just above the flare of the nostrils	Governs the sense of smell, the sinuses, and the ears. Alleviates sinus congestion due to colds or allergies.	Kapha
Vidhura marma	Behind and below each ear	Governs the sense of hearing. Decongests ear canals; reduces ringing in the ears; strengthens the neck.	Vata
Krikatika marma	The base of the skull, at the junction of the head and neck	Relieves tension headaches; increases circulation to the brain and clear thinking.	Kapha
Amsa marma	At the base of the neck on the trapezius muscles	Controls the fifth chakra (vishuddha, the throat chakra). Releases shoulder pain and back tension.	Pitta and vata
Hridaya marma	At the center of the sternum	Controls the fourth chakra (anahata, the heart chakra). Governs blood plasma and the circulatory system; boosts immunity.	Pitta
Brihati marma	On either edge of the scapulae close to the spine	Releases tension in the back, shoulders, and heart. Relieves excess heat.	Major pitta point

MARMA POINT	LOCATION*	THERAPEUTIC QUALITY	RELATED DOSHAS**
Nabhi marma	At the navel, around the belly button. This is a large point, four finger-widths in diameter.	Controls the third chakra (*manipura*, the navel chakra). Governs the small intestines. Main point for the digestive system and agni, the digestive fire.	Major pitta point
Basti marma	Between the pubic symphisis and the belly button in the hypogastric region	Governs the urinary and reproductive systems.	Vata
Kukundara marma	On either side of the sacrum, just above the fleshy part of the buttocks	Controls the second chakra (*svadhistahana*, the reproductive organs). Governs blood formation and the menstrual cycle.	Pitta
Guda marma	The perineum, at the base of the coccyx	Controls the first chakra (*muladhara*, the root chakra). Controls the execretory, urinary, reproductive, and menstrual systems.	Vata
Kurpara marma	At the elbow joint. This is a large point, three finger-widths in diameter.	Controls the liver and spleen, the blood, and the circulatory system.	Pitta
Kshipra marma	Located between the thumb and index finger. Also located between the first and second toes.	Tones the heart and lungs.	Pitta
Janu marma	The front point is located at the root of the knee; the back point is located behind the knee cap.	Tones the liver and spleen; lubricates the joints. Governs circulation to the legs.	Pitta
Gulpha marma	At the ankle joint, the sensitive area below the ankle bulge. Two finger-widths in diameter.	Relieves stiffness and leg fatigue; a natural pain reliever.	Tridoshic point
Talahridaya marma	Upper center of the sole in line with the third toe. Also located at the center of palm in line with third finger.	Stimulates the lungs and respiratory system.	Major kapha point

*Based on the research of Vamadeva (Dr. David Frawley).

**This column indicates which doshas benefit most from receiving pressure on that marma.

Apply pressure for approximately 5 to 10 seconds for general upkeep, or for up to one minute for deeper therapy. In order to prevent injury or discomfort, make sure to use the pad of the thumb. Direct pressure or circular motion can be applied, followed by a gentle massage of the region.

Clockwise motion is strengthening and helps to revitalize a marma point while counterclockwise movement helps to remove blockage and stagnation. But when considering clockwise or counterclockwise movement, don't overanalyze your work!

As you work on the marmas, visualize each point as an essential transfer station that passes vital energy throughout the region. Encourage the free and peaceful flow of energy through each transfer point. Direct your own breathing to the marma point, inhaling positive healing energy and exhaling negativity and tension. You may also direct your recipient to breathe into a marma point that seems particularly tender or stagnant.

When experiencing marma pressure your client may feel a range of sensations—a delicious sense of release, a stimulation of energy, or a sense of lightness directly following the removal of pressure. If your client experiences pain while you are working on a particular marma, there may be a blockage or stagnant energy occurring at that point. In such cases, only work as deeply as your client is comfortable and do not cause excessive discomfort.

Never work on the marma points on a client who is pregnant, diagnosed with cancer, or suffering from inflammation or a skin disorder. Points on the face, head, and abdomen are more sensitive, so apply less pressure to these areas. Points on the arms, legs, feet, and hands are easiest to work on and can be very powerful in their effects.

In order to maintain the even distribution of energy, be sure to massage the marma points on both the right and left sides of the body. When working on marmas with multiple locations, such as the kshipra point, located on the hands and feet, make sure to massage both the lower and the upper points to prevent an imbalance of energy.

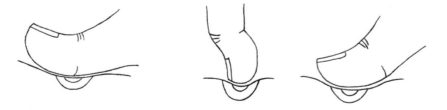

Proper use of the thumbs is important. Hyperextension (left) can lead to thumb injury. Applying pressure with the tip of the thumb (center) can cause discomfort for the recipient. Use the pad of the thumb (right) when applying pressure to the marma points.

MARMA APPROACH FOR EACH DOSHA

Whether the points are worked during energy-line palpation or are massaged separately at the end of the treatment, there are some general methods for customizing this aspect of the massage according to the doshic needs of each client.

When applying the appropriate massage style for a given dosha, whether it be sattvic, rajasic, or tamasic, the practitioner effectively becomes a conduit of universal energy and embodies the qualities of that guna. Of all the massage techniques a practitioner can apply, the most important is *intention*. It is important to take the time to willfully connect to the appropriate approach before beginning a session and to maintain that approach throughout the massage.

Embodying a quality or energetic force when giving a massage is a powerful process that must be done with mindful awareness in order to avoid disturbing the practitioner's own doshic balance. Practitioners can maintain a certain level of neutrality and egolessness by remembering that, in giving a Thai Yoga Massage based on the principles of Ayurveda, we are offering ourselves as vehicles for transmitting sacred wisdom teachings about the body that are both ancient and effective. When we remove interference from the ego, the intuitive energy of the universe can flow through us unimpeded.

Taking the Namaskar position at the beginning and end of each session serves as a reminder to attune ourselves to this universal energy that expands beyond the self. A pleasant-sounding bell or the sound of *Om* serves to bring closure to a session and to reestablish the physical and energetic separation between practitioner and recipient.

Despite the doshic variances among your clientele, it is recommended that you begin your massage with a sattvic touch to relax the recipient's body before applying a more rigorous approach.

Customizing sen energy-line work according to a client's dosha requires adapting your working pace and pressure to provide the recommended rhythm for that dosha. Kaphas require the most rapid pace for sen-line work, with a recommended pause of one second during palming and thumbing. A moderate pace with light pressure and an approximate pause of two seconds during palming and thumbing is most beneficial for pittas. When receiving palming or thumbing along the sen lines, vatas benefit from a slower pace. A three-second pause before the practitioner changes hands would be appropriate for vata recipients, who need to be reminded to slow down and embrace moments of stillness.

Because the approximate time allotted to sen work during a massage should be equivalent for all three doshas, one must adjust the distance and speed of rounds to the chosen pace. This adjustment follows basic common sense, but is good to consider before performing a massage. For example, when doing sen-line work on a vata client the recommended slow vata rhythm can be offset by placing our palms

SEN-LINE WORK FOR EACH DOSHA

VATA	Meditative rhythm, with slow pacing and moderate pressure to increase regularity and promote circulation and deep breathing. Hold: Pause for 3 seconds before alternating hands during palming or thumbing.
PITTA	Cooling approach that does not overstimulate blood circulation or irritate sensitive pitta skin. Moderate pacing and pressure. Hold: Pause for 2 seconds before alternating hands during palming or thumbing.
KAPHA	Energizing rhythm and firm pressure to remove stagnation and increase circulation. Hold: Pause for 1 second before changing hands during palming or thumbing.

a greater distance away from each other. Kapha types, on the other hand, require a more vigorous pacing which can be offset by less distance between our palms. Again, this will require more thought at the beginning, but should become a natural exercise as your understanding of Ayurveda deepens.

Our journey has so far uncovered several tools for customizing a Thai Yoga Massage session according to the Ayurvedic constitution of our clients. We will now look at how we can direct our breath and the breath of our clients as a final therapeutic component to Thai Yoga Massage.

Thai Massage Pranayama

The essence of all healing is to increase prana, the vital force that makes life possible. This subtle form of energy is obtained through air, food, water, sunlight, correct breathing, yoga asanas, and the compression and release of massage. A lack of touch or love can lead to a lack of prana, while a nurturing massage or bodywork session can increase and restore prana. A person can also regulate the intake of prana through deep yogic breathing and pranayama breath exercises.

When awakened, prana becomes a powerful tool for healing and consciousness that can strengthen a bodywork practice. Bodywork practitioners with high levels of prana have a greater capacity to heal others without risking depleting their own energy sources.

Within the Lotus Palm method of Thai Yoga Massage we teach several breath techniques that increase the pranic potentials of our work and simultaneously help to restore our own pranic reserves. When combined with Ayurveda, these breathing techniques emerge as essential ingredients for bringing doshic harmony to our clients and ourselves. (For those familiar with Kam Thye's first book, the following material also appeared in *Thai Yoga Massage*.)

BREATHING TECHNIQUES

Let's begin by looking at six breathing techniques taught at the Lotus Palm School of Thai Yoga Massage and consider which dosha most benefits from each method. This will be followed by a review of some easy and effective breathing exercises that one can practice during a massage session, in a yoga class, or at home.

Mindful Breathing

Mindful breathing is closely associated with the meditative state in Thai Yoga Massage. Mindful breathing is a meditation in motion, with the practitioner observing his breath from moment to moment as the dance of the massage unfolds. In this way the practitioner is fully focused on the work with the recipient. Mindful breathing, the most commonly used breath technique in a Thai Yoga Massage session, benefits all three doshas.

Synchronized Breathing

In synchronized breathing the practitioner is attentive to the recipient's breath, following the recipient's breath at first and then gradually enticing both breaths into a steady rhythm. This technique is mainly used when massaging the abdominal region. This tender area of the body houses many of our vital organs. When the practitioner marries a therapeutic touch with the breath, the result can be a very soothing, calming experience for the recipient. This breathing technique is most suitable for vata and pitta recipients.

Directed Breathing

With directed breathing the practitioner indicates to the recipient when to inhale and when to exhale, the breath matching different stages of a posture or stretch. For example, in the Demi Lotus the practitioner asks the recipient to inhale before performing the posture and then directs her to exhale as she is brought into a deeper pose. This technique is useful in enabling the practitioner to give the recipient a deeper stretch and generally results in a good release of tension from the body.

Directed breathing is most suitable for deep stretches that occur in multiple stages, such as Lunar Stretch, Demi Lotus, or Cobra. The practitioner directs the client to inhale, in preparation for the pose; he then directs her to exhale as he brings her into the deepest portion of the stretch. This exhilarating breath technique is great for engaging your kapha recipients. A gentle and nurturing version of the directed breath can also benefit vatas, who often forget to breathe!

Double Breathing

In double breathing the practitioner follows the directed breathing technique, then repeats it a second time for a deeper opening. For example, in Shiva Twist the practitioner directs the recipient to inhale, and then moves her into the twist as she exhales. The practitioner then holds the posture and asks the recipient to take a second deep breath, then moves into a deeper thoracic twist during the exhalation.

This technique is most suitable for postures that work on the back. Double breathing provides a pranic energy boost and promotes an invigorating stretch that is most suitable for kapha recipients.

Induced Breathing

When practicing induced breathing, the practitioner follows the recipient's exhalation and then gradually applies pressure to the body, forcing a deeper release of the breath. This technique is mainly used while working on the back, an area of the body that can carry a lot of tension.

Awareness of the breath is not always evident in the back; a forceful exhalation brings an inhalation full of awareness to any area of the back that has been compressed. This encourages a great release of tension, as it is very comforting to remain inactive as a recipient and be brought into a breath. This passive experience of letting go is particularly good for our pitta clients, who often have trouble relinquishing control, even during a massage.

Cooling Breathing

The cooling breathing technique can be useful when working on a high pitta client or during the hot summer months. This breath is a form of directed breathing that is done through the mouth and can be a useful counterbalance to heating postures, such as strong backbends. For example, once you have placed your recipient into Cobra pose, direct her to inhale and exhale through the mouth.

This cooling breath is a wonderful tool for helping pitta clients release excess heat in the body and mind, which may be released in the form of a sigh.

For those familiar with the *sithali* breath exercise (see page 79), you may guide your client to use this yogic breathing technique during a posture. For example, after pulling your client up into the Udana stretch, instruct her to take three sithali breaths before lowering her arms. This breathing technique is most appropriate for pitta clients, and for the other body types in the hot summer months.

There are a few points to bear in mind when practicing breathing techniques in Thai Yoga Massage. It can be intrusive for the practitioner to overmanipulate the recipient's breath. Likewise, strong, noisy breathing, as if somebody is breathing close to the ear, can disturb the recipient's state of rest. In this situation the recipient can be led into synchronizing his or her breath with the practitioner's, which is unnecessary.

Keep in mind that in a Thai Yoga Massage session the recipient is in a passive state and the practitioner is active, producing a very different breath rhythm for each. As well, each person's lung capacity is different. Don't feel that you are in a rush during a session and go chasing after the recipient's breath. Notice if you begin to enter a panting breath rhythm, which can disturb the client and cause you to overheat. Staying mindful will allow a gentle rhythm to emerge between you.

BREATH APPROACH FOR EACH DOSHA

Now that we have considered the main breath techniques used in Thai Yoga Massage and some tips for integrating breathwork into a massage, let's consider the breathing approaches most suitable for each dosha. If you are not familiar with all of the breathing techniques mentioned here, please refer to a yoga book or an experienced yoga teacher for further instructions.

Vata Approach to Breath

The irregular and anxious nature of vatas is commonly revealed in a shallow and inconsistent breath. Listen carefully to your recipient; if you notice that she hasn't breathed for a while, it is very likely that she is a vata person, or at the very least is experiencing a vata imbalance. In such cases, the directed breathing technique is ideal for reminding your vata recipients to breathe consistently and deeply.

Use a nurturing approach and direct the recipient to take steady, consistent, and calming breaths to help release emotional tension. This is particularly useful when executing forward bends, which are restorative and vata-reducing by nature. Ask the recipient to inhale deeply and then exhale completely as you apply light pressure to stabilize and release her forward.

Synchronized breath is another Thai Yoga Massage breathing technique that benefits vata individuals. If you maintain steady, consistent, and calming breaths, your recipient will likely follow suit. But do make sure to breathe quietly and naturally to avoid disturbing your easily distracted vata recipients.

Pranayama, or breathing exercises, can be an excellent way of revitalizing the body and achieving greater mental clarity. Of all three body types, vata individuals most require a regular pranayama practice to relieve anxiety and restore energy. Remember that vata is made up of air and ether; by regulating the breath we are working directly with the vata dosha.

We can help our high-vata recipients by recommending a few basic breathing exercises for their own home practice. One of the best pranayama exercises to reduce vata nervousness is deep yogic breathing into the abdomen. You can demonstrate this exercise to your recipient by lying on your back with your hands gently interlaced on the abdomen, just below the navel. As you inhale, the diaphragm expands to massage the abdominal organs, lifting the abdomen so that your fingers gently separate. When you exhale your hands release as your diaphragm moves down, pushing all of the stale air out of the lungs and abdomen. Individuals with vitiated vata should practice this breathing technique for at least five to ten minutes daily in combination with the vata yoga exercises outlined in chapter 15.

Another effective yogic breathing technique for vata individuals is anuloma viloma, or alternate nostril breathing. This practice regulates breathing through the right and left nostrils and thereby balances the pingala (or solar) nadi and the ida (or lunar) nadi. This exercise balances the heating and cooling energies of the body and increases the absorption of prana in the head and senses.

Pitta Breath Approach

When directed properly, breathing can also be a formidable method of countering high pitta and reducing excessive heat. During a Thai Yoga Massage session the breath techniques that most benefit pitta recipients are synchronized breathing, cooling breathing, and induced breathing. By synchronizing your breath with the client's and gradually slowing down the breath rhythm, you are gradually cooling down the body. In cases of overheating or burning sensations, direct the recipient to practice cooling breathing by breathing through the mouth.

Very often a pitta recipient has trouble sitting back and passively enjoying a massage—they may even help you execute many of the postures! If you notice this happening, the induced breathing technique can gently encourage pitta recipients to let go of control.

For home practice, there are several cooling pranayama exercises that will help to alleviate excess pitta. The technique of sithali involves curling the sides of the tongue to make a straw for "sipping" the air as you inhale. Close the mouth and hold the breath for a few seconds before exhaling through the nose. For *sitkari,* a similar technique that is beneficial for those who might find the sithali breath difficult, press the tip of the tongue against the upper palate to expose the back of the tongue. As you inhale deeply, a hissing sound occurs; then close your mouth and retain the breath as long as possible. Exhale quietly through the nose.

Direct your client to repeat either of these cooling exercises five to ten times in one sitting.

Kapha Breath Approach

Pranayama is a very effective tool for relieving the excessive phlegm or mental stagnation that may effect kaphas. When working on a kapha person, the best breathing techniques to apply are induced breathing and double breathing. The induced breathing technique encourages a deep and complete exhalation, emptying the lower and upper lungs and clearing out the respiratory system. In the double breathing technique, the recipient takes an exhilarating breath to deepen a stretch and wake up the body and mind. In cases of stagnant or sluggish kapha, rapid breaths can be encouraged to maintain energy and heat

BREATH APPROACH FOR EACH DOSHA

VATA

Breath approach	Quiet, nourishing, regular; deep abdominal breathing
During the massage	Directed breath, synchronized breath (with abdominal massage)
Home techniques	Deep breathing into the abdomen
	Anuloma viloma (alternate nostril breathing)

PITTA

Breath approach	Relaxed, quiet breaths that cool the body and mind
During the massage	In cases of overheating or burning sensations, direct the recipient to exhale through the mouth
	Cooling breath, synchronized breath
Home techniques	Sithali
	Sitkari

KAPHA

Breath approach	Exhilarating, energizing, heating
During the massage	Double breath, induced breath
Home techniques	Kapalabhati: rapid pumping breaths through the abdomen
	Brahmari: Humming breath

throughout a session. This also warms up the body and increases circulation, promoting positive regeneration.

There are several pranayama exercises that break up excessive phlegm and increase alertness as part of a kapha home practice. *Kapalabhati* is a rapid pumping breath exercise in which the abdomen is actively contracted in a series of quick exhalations. During this technique the diaphragm rises, forcing air out of the lungs and clearing the respiratory system to loosen mucus. Another beneficial pranayama practice for kapha individuals is *brahmari,* or humming breath. To execute this technique, make a snoring sound as you inhale, vibrating the throat area. On the exhale make a humming sound that resembles a bee and extend your exhalation as long as possible.

THE PRACTICE SECTION TO COME

The following chapters will take you through a Thai Yoga Massage series that will allow you to customize your massage practice according to the Ayurvedic needs of your recipients. The Ayurvedic quality of each posture is clearly outlined and is followed by an "Ayurvedic tip," which provides practical and easy-to-use guidelines on effectively integrating this art into your practice. A reference to the vayus being activated in each posture is also provided.

The Ayurvedic symbol next to each posture provides a quick and straightforward reference to the doshic quality of each posture. The **V P K** ▲ symbol is used for exercises that balance all three doshas. This would apply to neutralizing postures, such as Namaskar. Arrows pointing downward (↓) indicate that a posture reduces a particular dosha; for example V↓ shows that that particular posture lowers vata, and would therefore benefit a vata person. Arrows pointing upward (↑) indicate that a posture increases a particular dosha and so would be less beneficial for someone of that constitution. The number of arrows reflects the degree that the dosha is increased or decreased. The instructions for the Palming Shoulders posture carries the symbol V↓↓↓ P↓↓ K↑↑, for example. This means that it strongly reduces vata (due to its grounding effect) and is therefore most beneficial for a vata person. The posture is also good for pitta types, but would be less beneficial for kaphas due to its stabilizing nature.

Each of the eighteen key marma points discussed in chapter 6 are worked on in this massage series. The postures have been carefully selected and sequenced to create a balanced tridoshic series that is beneficial for all three doshas. Like a well-designed yoga class, this series provides counterstretches to backbends, forward bends, and twists.

This series has also been designed to incorporate the six fundamental movements of the spine: flexion, extension, flexion to the right and left, and rotation to the right and left. Special care has been taken to provide alternatives to the frequent use of palms

THE AYURVEDIC SYMBOLS LEGEND

V P K ▲	Tridoshic, balanced		
↓↓↓	Strongly reduces	↑↑↑	Strongly increases
↓↓	Reduces	↑↑	Increases
↓	Reduces slightly	↑	Increases slightly

and thumbs in Thai Yoga Massage; included are techniques that integrate the use of the elbows, knees, and forearms in applying pressure to the recipient's body. Finally, the medical benefits of each posture are outlined, as are important precautions and useful adaptations.

The chapters and postures are organized in accordance with the structure of a full-body Thai Yoga Massage, and are presented according to two levels of massage: basic and extended. A basic session lasts approximately one hour and includes all poses in the chapter with the exception of those with the symbol †. For an extended session of approximately two-and-a-half hours, include the postures indicated by the symbol †. The session begins with the sitting postures and then moves on to double- and single-foot exercises, sen work on the legs, and single-leg exercises. These are followed by the back-position postures and double-leg exercises. The session finishes with a restful massage of the abdomen, chest, arms, hands, and face.

Before beginning the massage, take the time to assess your recipient's predominant dosha using the Ayurvedic constitutional text on pages 195 to 197. At least thirty minutes will be needed to fill out the questionnaire and answer any questions that may arise.

Review the massage approaches presented in chapter 3 and integrate the appropriate pace, pressure, holds, breathing, essential oils, and incense to suit each recipient's unique needs. By familiarizing yourself with the Ayurvedic quality of the postures you can apply those poses and touch techniques that most benefit your client. This does not mean that you need to memorize the exact Ayurvedic symbol provided for each posture. Do become familiar with the general rules governing movement and energy flow, and then drop your analytical mind and let your intuition guide your work in the session. You can come back to these pages after a session and integrate the knowledge that you have picked up through your hands and your senses with the information you are assimilating from the book.

Finally, there's a saying that goes "no pain no gain." However, in the practice of Thai Yoga Massage this is not the case. It is very important to respect the recipient's physical limitations and pain threshold. Thai Yoga Massage is a firm and dynamic therapy;

however, it should not be torturous to the recipient. Regardless of a person's doshic type, always remember to respect, listen, and request feedback.

As we ready ourselves to explore the Thai Yoga Massage practice presented in the next chapters, let us take a moment to meditate on the Buddhist spirit of *metta,* unconditional love for all beings. As a physical application of loving-kindness in action, Thai Yoga Massage has the ability to operate at the highest level of healing. In order to truly practice these arts at the highest level, we must cultivate the seed of metta within our own hearts and those around us. By listening to the needs of others in our daily lives, we strengthen our intuitive skills of awareness and the universal connectiveness of all beings. In this way Thai Yoga Therapy emerges as a vehicle for self-knowledge and transformation.

Have a good practice. Namaste.

PART 3
❖❖
The Thai Yoga
Massage Series

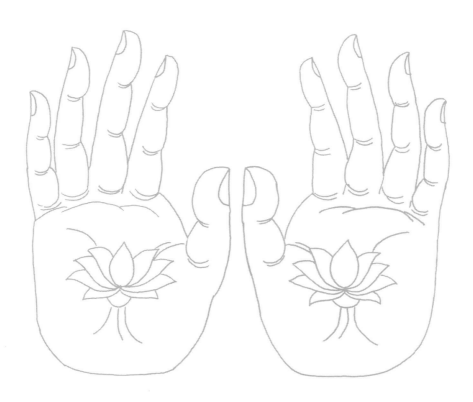

Sitting Postures

Once you have assessed the Ayurvedic constitution of your recipient and created the appropriate massage environment, you are ready to begin the Thai Yoga Massage session. We begin with the sitting positions to open the upper body and to address the shoulders, an area of the body where much stress can accumulate. Here you will set the tone and atmosphere for the entire session, so take the time to draw your energy to the journey on which you are about to embark.

Before beginning, consciously transform yourself into a vehicle of Ayurvedic healing by embodying the appropriate qualities that are most beneficial for your recipient. When working on a high-vata recipient, embody qualities of stability and warmth in order to ground vata anxiety and worry. In the case of pitta recipients, act as a vehicle of cooling and "sweet" energy to calm and diffuse any anger and frustration they may be experiencing. For kapha recipients, embody an energetic approach in order to break up kapha stagnation and inertia.

During the sitting postures, listen with your hands and rub, squeeze, and soothe any tense areas that you discover. Do not use jerky movements; especially avoid the infamous maneuver of cracking the neck.

Thai Yoga Massage begins with the centering and meditative posture of Namaskar, the traditional Indian and Thai greeting that symbolizes respect, inner peace, and purity of the heart. By joining the hands in front of the heart prior to beginning the massage, the practitioner creates a healing space of metta, or loving-kindness and compassion.

In performing this simple gesture the practitioner communicates the profound message, "I bow to the Divine in you." This act reminds us of the importance of moment-to-moment awareness and of respecting and honoring the tradition of Thai Yoga Massage. It is also an ideal time to meditate on the appropriate Ayurvedic approach you will embody during the session.

Namaskar V P K ▲

Stand behind the recipient, who is comfortably seated either with legs crossed or legs extended. The recipient's hands should be resting on her knees.

Join your palms together in front of the heart (**fig. 8.1**). Keep the eyes closed softly for a few moments and call to mind the appropriate Ayurvedic massage approach for your recipient. Take several quiet breaths reflecting on those qualities that you will embody to balance your recipient's predominant dosha.

Adaptation: If the recipient is uncomfortable sitting on the mat, you can invite her to sit on a pillow.

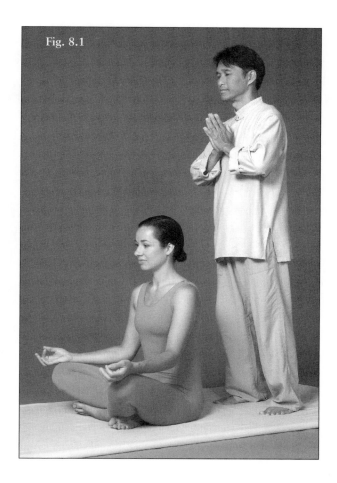

Fig. 8.1

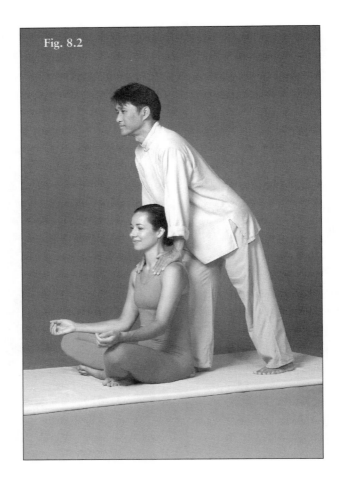

Fig. 8.2

Palming Shoulders V↓↓↓ P↓↓ K↑↑

Using the Tai Chi stance, support the recipient's back with the lateral side of your right lower leg (**fig. 8.2**). Note that the right heel is turned outward and the toes are turned slightly inward to make the fleshy part of the leg available to the recipient's back. Make sure the recipient is fully supported and her spine is aligned.

Place your palms on top of the recipient's shoulders, keep your arms and back straight, and lean your body weight into the recipient's shoulders. The point of contact is on the trapezius muscle, not the clavicle.

Use forward rock to palm the shoulders. The direction of pressure is straight down.

Adaptation: For comfort, a pillow can be placed between your lower leg and the recipient's back.

Benefits: Releases tension in the trapezius muscles; relieves knots (hypercontracted muscles); increases shoulder and neck mobility.

Precautions: Avoid pressing on bones (the clavicle and the humerus), as this can be painful.

Vayus activated: Apana, samana

Ayurvedic tip: The grounding compression on the shoulders in this posture makes it ideal for vatas. The airy, floating nature of vata is rooted downward, directing apana vayu downward.

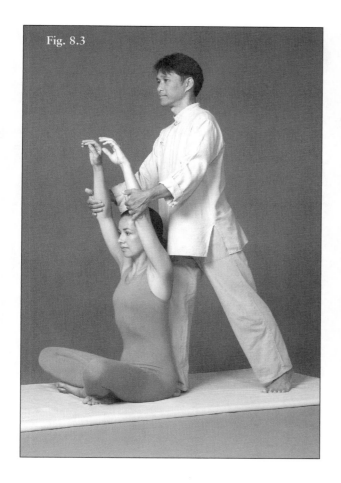

Fig. 8.3

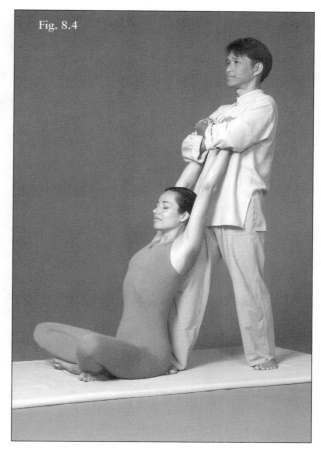

Fig. 8.4

Udana Stretch V↑ P↓ K↓↓

Remaining in Tai Chi stance, ask the recipient to raise her hands above her head. Cross your hands around her arms slightly below the elbows.

Glide your hands along her forearms (**fig. 8.3**) and interlock opposite palms with the recipient.

With your back straight, lean back and stretch the recipient's arms and shoulders upward (**fig. 8.4**). This creates an upward lift and awakening of udana vayu.

Benefits: Tractions the upper spine; tones the abdomen; increases mobility in the shoulders; stretches the subscapularis muscles; increases lung capacity; relieves congestion and tightness in the chest.

Precautions: Avoid this posture if the recipient has a history of frozen shoulder or dislocation, as this could cause discomfort.

Vayus activated: Udana, prana

Ayurvedic tip: Use this posture to awaken your kapha recipients, but avoid in people with high vata.

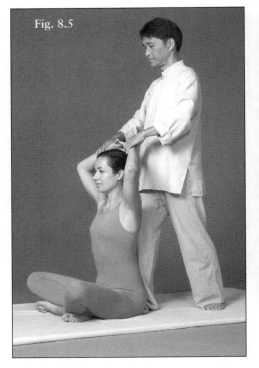

Fig. 8.5

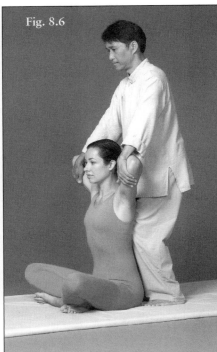

Fig. 8.6

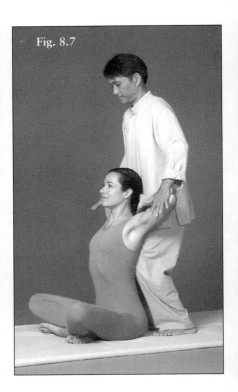

Fig. 8.7

✝ Butterfly Knee V↑ P↓↓ K↓↓↓

From Udana Stretch, place the recipient's hands at the back of her head and ask her to interlace her fingers (**fig. 8.5**).

Bring your left leg forward to stand with feet shoulder-width apart, your knees high up on the recipient's scapulae; place your hands on the recipient's upper arms (**fig. 8.6**). Bend your knees as you lift the arms upward and slightly backward, extending the recipient's upper spine (**fig 8.7**). Repeat this last step three times.

This is a nice chest opener.

Adaptation: Place a cushion between your knees and the recipient's scapulae for added comfort.

Benefits: Creates thoracic expansion; awakens the senses; energizes the body; promotes deep breathing.

Precautions: Place your knees high up on the scapulae, along the paravertebral muscles, to avoid pinching the middle back. Avoid putting pressure on the spine. Take extreme care when working on a recipient with previous shoulder dislocation.

Vayus activated: Udana, prana

Ayurvedic tip: This posture opens the chest, relieves congestion, and promotes an upward movement that awakens the senses. It is a great energy boost for kaphas.

Lunar Stretch V↑ P↓↓ K↓↓↓

Rest your hands on the recipient's upper back and ask her to interlace her fingers behind her head.

Kneel down in Open Archer stance, your right knee resting on the recipient's right hip (**fig. 8.8**).

Place your left hand on the recipient's left elbow and your right hand on her right elbow. Gently guide the recipient to rest her body weight onto your right thigh, providing a lengthening side stretch (**fig. 8.9**).

Bring your right hand to hold her left elbow; palm up and down the triceps muscles using your left hand (**fig. 8.10**). You can guide the elbow toward you to provide a gentle spinal rotation.

Repeat on the other side.

Benefits: Laterally flexes the spine; tones the spinal nerves, abdominal organs, and waist; increases peristalsis of bowels; stimulates agni, the digestive fire.

Vayus activated: Vyana, udana

Ayurvedic tip: This is another great chest opener for kaphas. Go gently with your vata recipients!

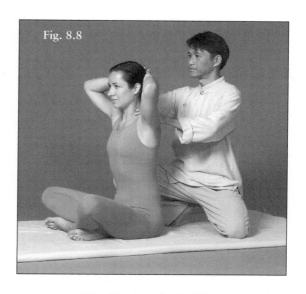

Fig. 8.8

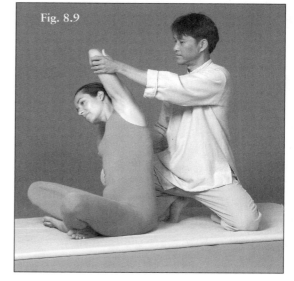

Fig. 8.9

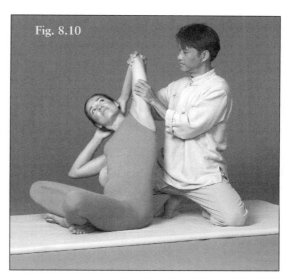

Fig. 8.10

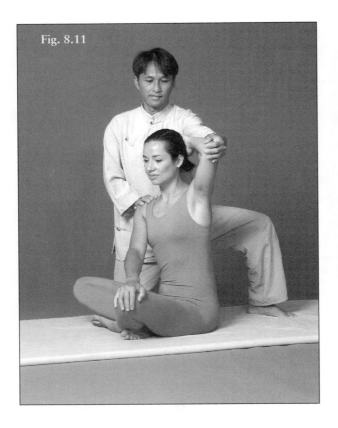

Fig. 8.11

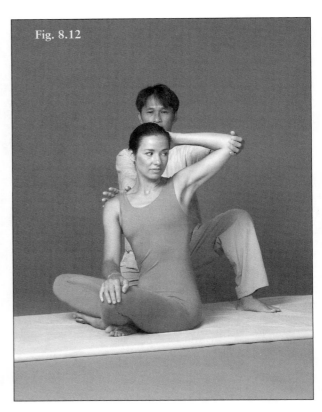

Fig. 8.12

Shiva Twist V↓↓ P↓ K↓↓↓

Finish Lunar Stretch with the recipient sitting vertically, spine aligned. Ask the recipient to release her right arm; place the right hand on her left knee. Scoop back and lift your left knee into Warrior stance so that you are perpendicular to your recipient. Place your right hand on her right shoulder and your left hand on her left elbow (**fig. 8.11**).

Sit back on your right heel, then push with your right hand and pull with your left to create a mid-thoracic rotation (**fig. 8.12**). Continue with the Shakti Twist on the right side (see instructions on the facing page) before repeating both twists on the other side.

Benefits: Stretches the pectoral muscles; opens the chest and encourages deep breathing; nour-

ishes the intervertebral disks; increases mobility and flexibility in the thoracic and lumbar spine; stretches and lengthens the sympathetic nerve chain; stimulates the digestive fire; releases toxins from the liver and spleen.

Precaution: Make sure your recipient's spine is in an upright position to avoid a clumsy and uncomfortable twist. With pregnant women, limit the twist to the upper thoracic region.

Vayus activated: Vyana, samana

Ayurvedic tip: All spinal rotations are tridoshic in nature, but the heating and energizing qualities of this twist makes it best for vata and kapha. Shiva is a Hindu god related to fire and masculine energy.

Shakti Twist V↓↓↓ P↓↓↓ K↓

From Shiva Twist, lift back up into Warrior stance as you place the recipient's left hand on her right shoulder.

Glide forward in your Warrior stance so that your right knee is close to the recipient's spine (**fig. 8.13**). Hold on to the recipient's left elbow with your right hand; place your left hand on her left scapula (**fig. 8.14**).

Pivot your body so that your left knee is resting on the recipient's left thigh as you gently pull with your right hand and push with your left (**fig. 8.15**). This intensifies the rotation and provides a counter-exercise to the Shiva Twist.

Repeat Shiva Twist to the right and Shakti Twist to the left before proceeding with the next posture.

When you finish, cup the recipient's right elbow and release her arm onto her lap. Center yourself behind her in Open Diamond stance.

Benefits: Compresses the pectoral muscles; stretches the rhomboid and levator scapulae muscles; nourishes the intervertebral disks and increases mobility and flexibility in the middle back; stimulates the digestive fire (agni) and releases toxins (ama) in the liver and spleen.

Precautions: Do not use jerky or fast movements. Avoid this posture if the recipient has osteoporosis or spinal problems. For pregnant women, limit the rotation to the upper thoracic region.

Vayus activated: Samana, vyana

Ayurvedic tip: This nurturing, inwardly directed counterrotation to the Shiva Twist is good for vata and pitta. Shakti, the creative force within Vedic culture, represents female energy.

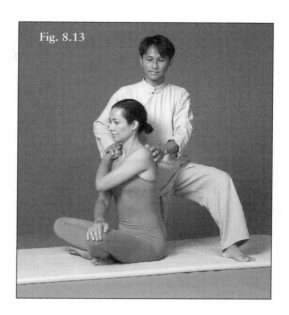
Fig. 8.13

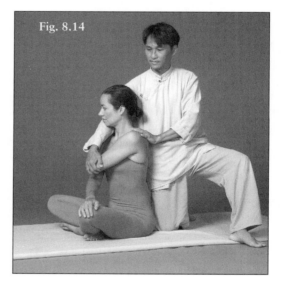
Fig. 8.14

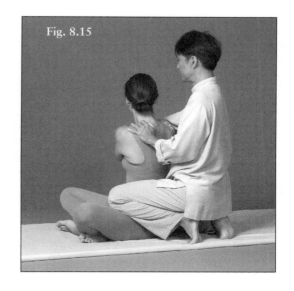
Fig. 8.15

✝ Whirlpool V↓↓ P↓↓ K↓↓

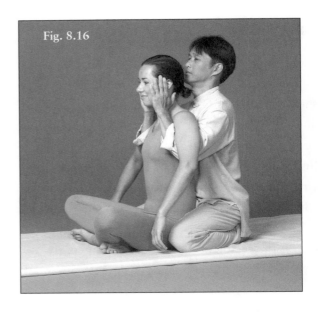

Fig. 8.16

After completing the Twist series on both sides, position your Open Diamond stance as close to the recipient as possible. Glide your forearms underneath her arms. Gradually lift your arms to place your palms on the sides of her head (**fig. 8.16**).

Staying steady in your pelvis, rotate your torso in whirlpool rock, using your body weight to encourage the recipient's body to roll with yours (**fig. 8.17**). Provide gentle traction through the neck as you lean back (**fig. 8.18**).

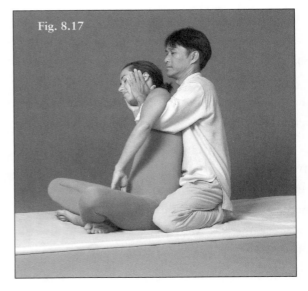

Fig. 8.17

Begin with small circles, gradually increasing the size of the rotation to complete five circles. Reverse the direction of your rotation to repeat on the other side.

Adaptation: A pillow can be placed between your chest and the recipient's back.

Benefits: Provides full spinal traction; mobilizes the vertebrae; increases circulation; massages the internal organs.

Precautions: Avoid with people with cervical spinal problems and osteoporosis, and the elderly.

Vayus activated: Vyana, prana

Ayurvedic tip: When performed gently this is a soothing pacifier for vata. Use a moderate pace for pitta and a more vigorous tempo for kapha.

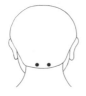

Krikatika Marma

This marma is located at the base of the skull on either side of the cervical spine. Working on this point helps to relieve tension headaches, increase circulation to the brain, and promote clear thinking. It is great for waking up kaphas!

Krikatika marma is stimulated during Whirlpool posture.

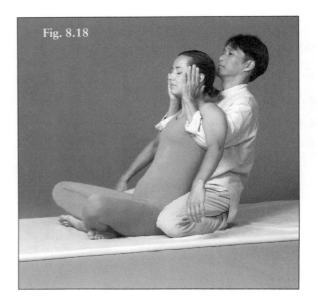

Fig. 8.18

† Table Top Twist V↓ P↓↓ K↓↓↓

From Whirlpool, lift up into Kneeling Diamond; place the recipient's hands behind her head and ask her to interlace her fingers (**fig. 8.19**).

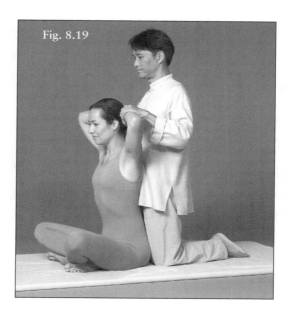

Fig. 8.19

Step into Warrior stance with your right foot in front of her crossed leg. Reach under her triceps and back through the triangles created by her bent arms, taking hold of her forearms. Bend her forward at the waist (**fig. 8.20**). The recipient's back should be flat, like a tabletop.

Keep your back straight as you gradually twist her torso to the left (**fig. 8.21**). Let this twist originate from your navel. Your right leg will straighten as you do this.

Repeat this twist once, then return to the center. Step into Warrior stance on the left side to repeat the Table Top Twist to the right.

Benefits: Provides upper lumbar spinal twist; stretches and twists the thoracic region; stretches the serratus anterior muscles; tones the kidneys.

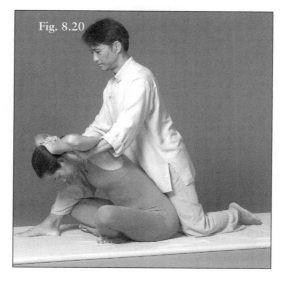

Fig. 8.20

Precaution: Avoid jerky movements and respect the limitations of your recipient. For pregnant women, limit the twist to the upper thoracic region.

Vayus activated: Vyana, prana

Ayurvedic tip: This dynamic twist is great for kaphas. It relieves tension in the upper back, where pittas tend to carry stress. Be careful with fragile vatas, as this stretch can be powerful.

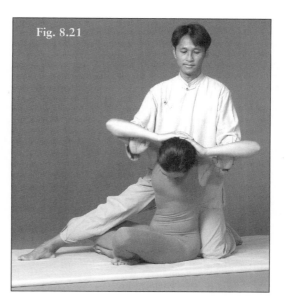

Fig. 8.21

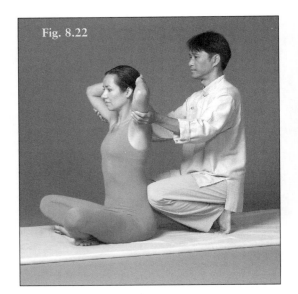

Fig. 8.22

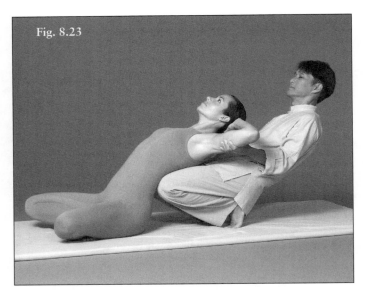

Fig. 8.23

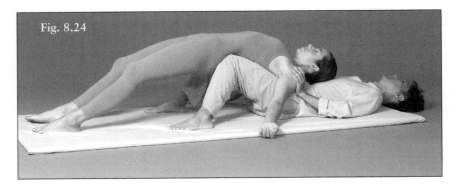

Fig. 8.24

✝ Bridge V↑↑ P↑ K↓↓↓

Finish Table Top Twist with the recipient sitting vertically, spine aligned and with hands interlaced. Come into a squat behind your recipient, shifting your hands to grasp her upper arms. Place your knees on either side of her spine on her low back (**fig. 8.22**).

Gradually lean back, allowing the recipient's weight to rest onto your lower body (**fig. 8.23**). Instruct the recipient to unfold her or his legs (**fig. 8.24**).

Rest your hands on the recipient's shoulders. Allow your recipient to relax in this position for three to five breaths (**fig. 8.25**).

To release, push into the recipient's shoulders to lift both of you into a sitting position (**fig. 8.26**). Cross your legs and rock forward to come into Warrior stance on the left side, in preparation for Forward Bend.

Before performing Bridge pose make sure to receive permission from your client, as this is a rigorous posture. Just before entering the pose, inform the recipient that you will be bringing her into a backbend; ask for feedback before you transition to the next posture. If there is some lower back discomfort, encourage the recipient to take a few deep breaths before proceeding.

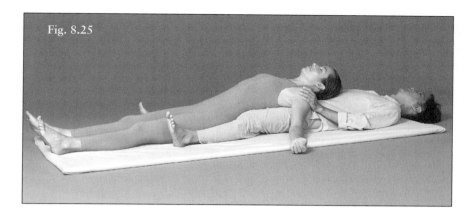

Fig. 8.25

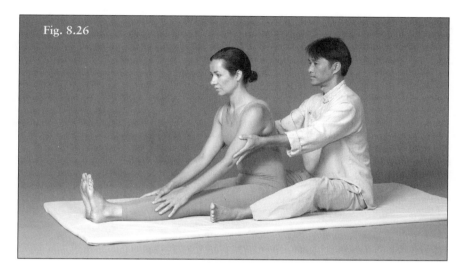

Fig. 8.26

Adaptation: If you have bony knees, place a cushion between your knees and the recipient's back.

Benefits: Extends the lumbar spine; opens and energizes the chest.

Precaution: In order to avoid the possibility of back strain, before executing the pose ask your recipient to extend his or her legs at the halfway point of the movement. Avoid doing this posture with people heavier than you and those with low back pain.

Vayus activated: Vyana, udana

Ayurvedic tip: Kaphas benefit greatly from this heating, dynamic backbend and chest opener. If you or your client has a bony vata frame, make sure to use a pillow between knees and back!

Forward Bend V↓↓↓ P↓↓↓ K↑↑

From Shakti Twist in the basic series or Bridge in the extended version, step forward into Warrior stance, left leg forward. Slide your hands up the recipient's arms to above the elbows and swing her forward so she bends at the waist, arms extended (**fig. 8.27**). This transition should be done in one fluid motion. Practice makes progress!

Using forward rock, palm up and down the paravertebral muscles, keeping your arms and back straight (**fig. 8.28**). For the chopping variation, press palms together and percuss into the recipient's back, making a "clapping" sound (**fig. 8.29**).

Adaptation: If the recipient does not have flexible hamstring muscles and is uncomfortable in Forward Bend, place a cushion between the legs and the abdomen.

Benefits: Relaxes and relieves back tension; provides a cooling counterstretch to Bridge pose.

Vayus activated: Prana, vyana

Ayurvedic tip: Forward bends are great for recharging vatas and can also relieve excess pitta heat. Forward bends tend to increase kapha. Instruct kapha recipients to keep palms on the floor with arms straight and chin up, to prevent collapsing through the chest.

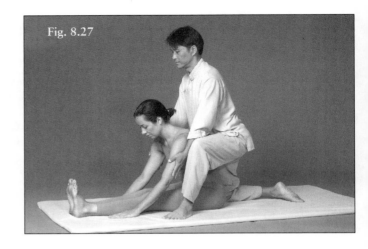

Fig. 8.27

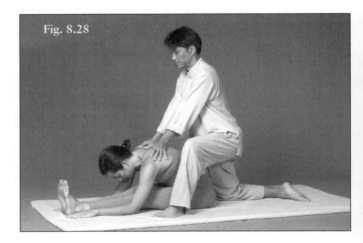

Fig. 8.28

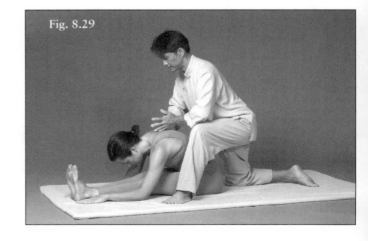

Fig. 8.29

Fish V↓ P↓↓ K↓↓↓

Place your hands on the recipient's shoulders and gently pull her up into sitting. Shift into Kneeling Diamond stance and cross your lower legs (**fig. 8.30**). Sit on the floor behind your crossed legs while holding onto the recipient's shoulders. Place your left hand on her shoulder and your right hand on her upper back (**fig. 8.31**).

Straighten your legs and place the balls of your feet on the recipient's low back. Pull gently backward with your right arm as you begin to gradually walk up the recipient's spine; in order to travel up the spine the practitioner must gracefully shuffle the buttocks backward. The recipient's torso and shoulders will begin to lower toward you; as the recipient falls toward you, you will naturally want to switch your hand positions so that the right arm is supporting the head and the left hand is supporting the back (**fig. 8.32**).

The Art of Thai Chopping

Chopping can be used to release and disperse tension in the back, shoulders, buttocks, thighs, and calves. Clients love it when done properly. However, this technique can be tricky, as your hands and fingers can easily slide out of place. Find the balance between soft and hard pressure in your hands. In the beginning your hands might not stay together and the sound may be weak and unimpressive. Do it a few hundred times and you will get it for sure! Chopping is a tridoshic technique that can be modified to your client's needs—it can be gentle and soothing for vatas; relaxing and dispersing for pittas, and stimulating and energizing for kaphas.

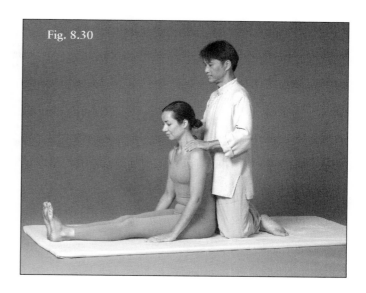

Fig. 8.30

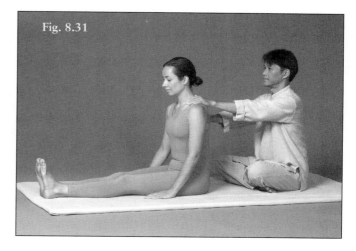

Fig. 8.31

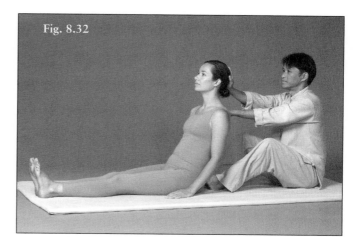

Fig. 8.32

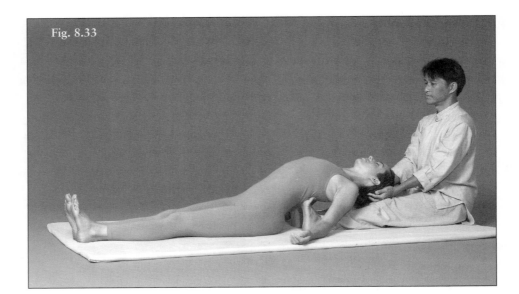

Fig. 8.33

Continue to support your recipient's downward arc as you travel up the spine with your feet. When the recipient reaches a full spinal extension, the balls of your feet will be at the midpoint of the scapulae and your legs will be straight (**fig. 8.33**).

Your toes will bend toward your head, as in Toe Arc stretch (see chapter 9, Double- and Single-Foot Postures). Allow the recipient's head to rest in your hands.

Benefits: Extends the upper back; releases tension in the thoracic spine and lumbar regions; opens the chest; relieves congestion and promotes deep yogic breathing; strengthens the thyroid and parathyroid; promotes blood flow to the brain.

Precaution: Make sure to support the recipient's head; if you don't you will exert excess pressure on the cervical spine, creating unnecessary (and potentially dangerous) hyperextension.

Common mistake: Practitioners do not keep their toes flexed, which is necessary for providing an effective upper-spine extension.

Vayus activated: Vyana, udana

Ayurvedic tip: Fish is a wonderful chest opener that relieves kapha congestion. It also expels excess heat from the body, as you are working on Brihati marma, a major pitta point.

Brihati Marma

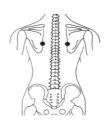

This point is located on the edge of either scapulae, close to the spine. This is a major pitta accumulation site; working on this point releases excess heat and blood.

Brihati marma is stimulated during Fish pose.

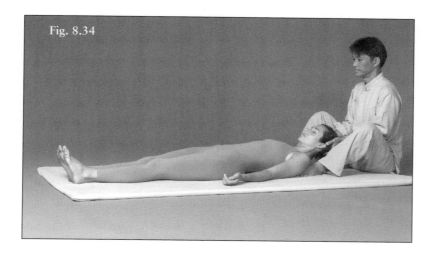

Fig. 8.34

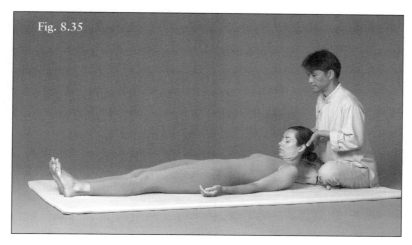

Fig. 8.35

Counter Fish V↓↓ P↓↓ K↑

To release Fish posture, continue to support the recipient's head with your hands as you lift your knees and place the soles of your feet on the mat (**fig. 8.34**). Gently move your legs into a cross-legged pose as you gradually lift and tuck the recipient's chin toward her chest (**fig. 8.35**).

Hold for three to five breaths to provide a good a counterstretch to Fish.

Benefits: Stretches the cervical spine and back of the neck as a counter to Fish posture; stimulates nerve endings at the base of the skull, improving functioning of sensory organs.

Precautions: Move slowly (even for kaphas!), as the back of the neck contains sensitive nerves, arteries, and veins. *Never* attempt cracking the neck, as this could lead to stroke or paralysis.

Vayus activated: Prana

Ayurvedic tip: A nice counter-exercise to Fish that draws the prana inward. In yoga this prana lock is called Jalandhara Bandha.

Amsa Pressure V P K ▲

From Counter Fish, rest the recipient's head on the mat. Place your thumb on the Amsa marma points, located in the middle of the trapezius muscle halfway between the shoulders and the neck (see box below).

With arms and back straight, forward rock to gradually apply thumb pressure on the Amsa marma (**fig. 8.36**). Sustain pressure for three to five breaths.

Benefits: Releases neck and shoulder tension.

Vayus activated: Apana, prana

Ayurvedic tip: To give a stronger massage to kapha recipients, apply pressure to each Amsa marma with your foot (**fig. 8.37**). Brace yourself by placing your arms behind you.

Transitional Flow

Stand up and walk to the recipient's feet in preparation for the double- and single-foot postures. Sit at the recipient's feet in Open Diamond stance.

We're now ready to move on to the Double- and Single-Foot Postures.

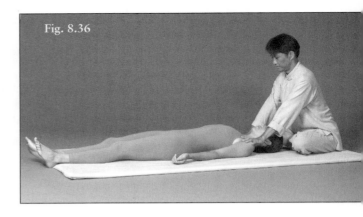

Fig. 8.36

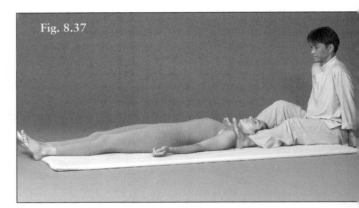

Fig. 8.37

Amsa Marma

This point is located in the middle of the trapezius muscle between the shoulders and neck. It controls the Vishuddha (throat) chakra, clears the chest, and promotes open communication.

Amsa marma is stimulated during the Amsa Pressure pose.

9

Double- and Single-Foot Postures

In the East there are many taboos surrounding the feet—where the feet can be pointed, whether they should be covered, and whose feet you are allowed to touch are all subjects of strong cultural proscriptions. In many cultures it is considered disrespectful to sit with your feet pointed at another person, and especially those who are highly revered. Yet a disciple may express devotion and love toward a guru by prostrating and touching, and sometimes even kissing, his or her feet. In certain parts of India, the earth that has been walked on by wise sages is considered purified.

Kam Thye experienced these traditions surrounding the feet firsthand while traveling in India many years ago, when he was welcomed with a cup of holy water used to wash a guru's feet. How could he say no to such a fast-track to enlightenment?!

In the double- and single-foot postures we honor our recipients by touching their feet, a gesture of respect and regard. The first three movements here work both feet simultaneously. Once you reach Mortar and Pestle, perform all the remaining movements on one foot and then switch to the other foot.

While working on this area of the body one may encounter the occupational hazard of unwelcome odors or dirty feet. My students often ask me what would be appropriate under these circumstances. I usually give them two answers. First, I tell them to work on the client's feet and then massage the face. Either you will lose the client, or the next time the client will return with pleasant smelling feet! Of course, this is only a joke. What I truly recommend is to always have a clean pair of socks on hand, just in case.

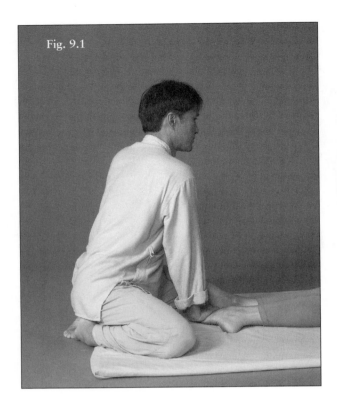

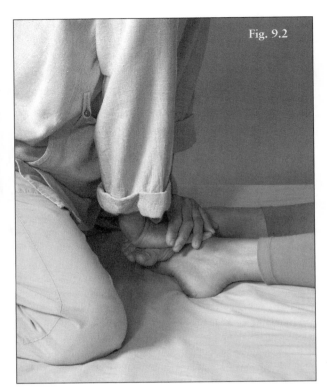

Foot Sandwich V↓↓ P↓↓ K↑

Sit in Open Diamond stance at the recipient's feet and position her legs shoulder-width apart. Place your right hand on top of the recipient's left foot. Gradually fold the foot toward the centerline, extending the sole toward the mat (**fig. 9.1**).

With your left hand, fold the recipient's right instep on top of her left foot.

Place both hands on her feet, palm over palm. Gradually rock forward, applying pressure as you maintain a firm hold (**fig. 9.2**). Repeat three times.

Repeat on the other side.

Benefits: Stretches the peroneus muscles; stimulates digestion by working on corresponding reflexology points; alleviates fatigue in the feet and legs; relieves symptoms of arthrosis and stiff ankles.

Precaution: Avoid in cases of foot injury or knee strain; do not press the ball of one foot directly onto the top of the other foot, as this can be painful.

Vayus activated: Samana, apana

Ayurvedic tip: For vatas, take extra care to avoid bone-to-bone contact. Apply stronger pressure to break up kapha stagnation.

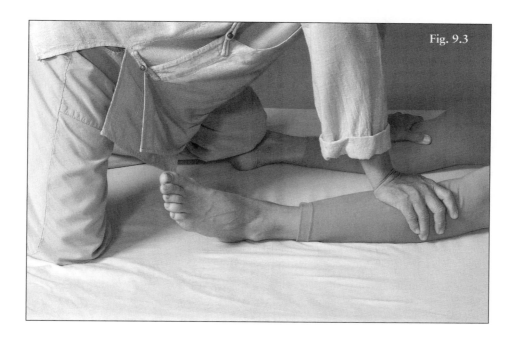

Fig. 9.3

✝ Kneeing Insteps V↓↓ P↓↓ K↓

In Open Diamond stance, position the recipient's feet shoulder-width apart. Place your palms on the recipient's lower legs and position your left knee on the recipient's right instep; rock forward (fig. 9.3). Apply gradual pressure as you knee up and down the instep, working on Sen Sumana. Repeat three times.

Switch knees and repeat on the other foot.

Benefits: Stretches and opens up the feet and the soleus muscles; tones the stomach, bladder, pancreas, and kidneys by working the corresponding reflexology points on the feet; alleviates fatigue in the feet and legs.

Precautions: Apply gradual knee pressure, as this massage can be intense. Distribute your body weight evenly between your hands and knees.

Vayus activated: Prana, vyana

Ayurvedic tip: All three types benefit from this exercise, as it activates movement along Sen Sumana, the main pathway for prana in the body. Apply strong pressure for kaphas.

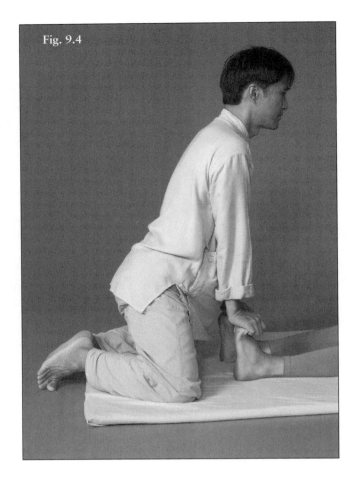

Fig. 9.4

Toe Arc V↓↓ P↓↓ K↓

Maintaining your Open Diamond stance, bring the recipient's feet into an upright position. Place your palms on the balls of her feet and rock forward, lifting up off your heels (**fig. 9.4**).

Arch the toes toward the recipient's head and maintain a steady hold. Release and repeat three times.

Benefits: Stretches the muscles on the soles of the feet; compresses the ankle joints; relieves tired legs and feet; relieves plantar fasciitis.

Precautions: Avoid this pose in cases of hyperextended knees or foot injuries.

Vayus activated: Vyana, apana

Ayurvedic tip: In this tridoshic exercise you are working on Sen Kalathari, a principal sen line that stimulates circulation and the removal of toxins.

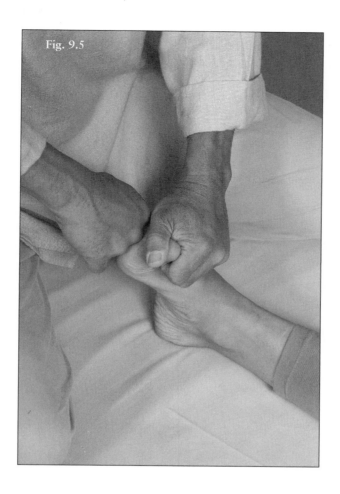

Fig. 9.5

✝ Mortar and Pestle V↓↓ P↓↓ K↓

From Toe Arc, center yourself in front of the recipient's right foot, sitting in Kneeling Diamond.

Use your left hand to arc the toes, exposing the area above the ball of the foot.

Make a fist with your right hand; rock forward and use your knuckles to massage the area at the base of the toes (**fig. 9.5**). Work from the big toe to the little toe. Repeat twice.

Benefits: Increases blood flow to the feet; relieves plantar fasciitis.

Vayus activated: Apana, vyana

Ayurvedic tip: This massage move flushes the toxins released in Toe Arc.

Gulpha Marma

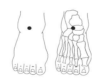

This point is located at the ankle joint, in the sensitive area just below the ankle bulge. It helps to relieve stiffness and leg fatigue. It is also a natural analgesic, or pain reliever.

Gulpha marma is stimulated during the Toe Arc.

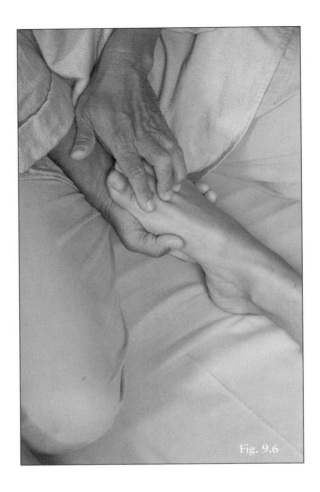

Fig. 9.6

✝ Shoe Polish V↓↓ P↓↓ K↓

From Mortar and Pestle, firmly hold the recipient's sole with your right hand.

Using the fingertips of your left hand, massage the top of her foot in a circular, spiraling motion. With a light whirlpool rock, work from the arch to the toes (**fig. 9.6**). Repeat five times.

Benefits: Increases circulation and lymphatic stimulation on the dorsal side of the foot.

Vayus activated: Apana, vyana

Ayurvedic tip: Your vata recipients will especially love this soothing, calming foot rub. Your kapha recipients may love it too much!

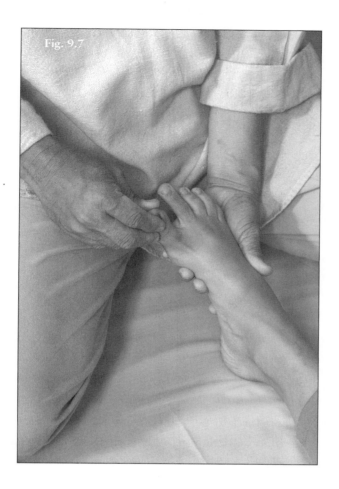

† Toe Dance V↓↓ P↓↓ K↓

From Shoe Polish, grasp the recipient's big toe by creating a clamp with your thumb, index finger, and middle finger.

Swirl the toe around, as though the toe is a delicate spoon with which you are stirring honey into hot tea (**fig. 9.7**). Complete three circles and then repeat in the other direction. Continue to work on all five toes in the same manner.

If you are giving an extended Thai Yoga Massage, return to the Mortar and Pestle and perform all the single-foot postures on the other foot. To end the foot exercises, caress all parts of the recipient's foot.

Benefits: Promotes circulation to the feet and toes; wakes up the toes.

Vayus activated: Apana, vyana

Ayurvedic tip: This a playful technique that can be especially good for dispersing pitta's intensity. Have fun with this swirling dance!

Transitional Flow

Move to the recipient's right side and take position in the Open Diamond stance. This is the end of the foot exercises.

We're now ready to move on to sen work on the legs and the single-leg postures.

10

Single-Leg Postures

We begin the single-leg postures by palming the sen lines on the legs to open the energy channels and increase blood circulation. This is followed by a single-leg *vinyasa*, or yoga flow, that includes several asana-based postures strung together with counter-stretches and complementary movements. The single-leg postures are often considered the most dynamic and challenging portion of the massage, as this flowing dance requires much practice and mastery over the working stances. But it is also considered the most fun—so enjoy!

When massaging the sen energy lines we are working directly with an individual's energetic life force, or prana. This form of pranic healing requires a great deal of mindfulness and subtle perception on the part of the practitioner. We must listen well with our hands, be aware of our recipient's body mechanics, and watch his or her face for signs of discomfort.

Begin by attuning yourself to the Ayurvedic constitution of your recipient and the natural quality of his or her energy flow. An easy way to do this is to consider the Ayurvedic analogy between the bodily pulse and the animals discussed in chapter 3. You may ask yourself: Does my recipient have quick and irregular vata energy that resembles a snake? Or is it more pitta in nature—strong and bounding like a frog? Or is it slow and graceful, like a kapha swan?

Once you are aware of the quality of your recipient's energy, follow the sen-line approach that most effectively harmonizes each constitution. Vata individuals benefit from a meditative, slow, and regular rhythm that helps to calm down and neutralize their erratic energy flow. A cooling approach with a moderate pace and pressure is most suitable for pittas. Kapha recipients will benefit from an energizing pace with strong pressure that breaks up physical and mental stagnation. For more details on each of these approaches, refer to chapter 3.

In Thai Yoga Massage there are three sen lines that run along the medial side of the leg and three that run along the lateral side. In this practice we focus on palming Sen Kalathari, which relieves leg fatigue and provides emotional balance.

We begin by working on the inner line of the left leg. Continue with palming the lateral side of the right leg, and then perform all of the single-leg poses on the right leg before walking around to repeat on the other side.

Palming Sen on Medial Side V P K ▲

Sit in Open Diamond stance alongside the recipient's right leg. Place your right hand on the inside of the recipient's left ankle and your left hand above the inside left knee (**fig. 10.1**).

Gradually palm the leg using Bamboo Rock, simultaneously moving from ankle to knee with your right hand and from knee to upper thigh with your left (**fig. 10.2**). Palm up and down the leg three times.

After completing this exercise, maintain your position to work on the lateral side of the right leg.

Benefits: Increases blood flow through the legs; removes waste materials through the venous and lymphatic systems; relieves muscular tension in legs and restless leg syndrome.

Vayus activated: Vyana, apana

Ayurvedic tip: Follow the appropriate massage approach for each dosha. For more details on this, see chapter 3.

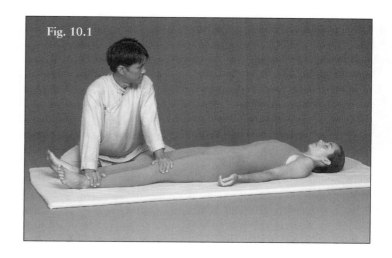
Fig. 10.1

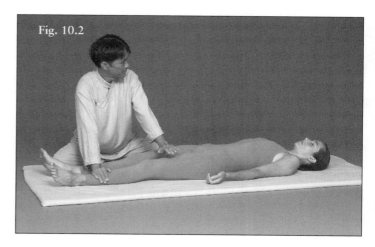
Fig. 10.2

Kneeing Sen on Lateral Side V↑ P↓ K↓↓↓

From Palming Sen on Medial Side, use your right hand to fold the recipient's right foot inward, exposing the tibialis anterior muscle.

Place your left palm on the recipient's outer right thigh and move into Open Archer stance so that your right knee is on the tibialis anterior muscle (**fig. 10.3**).

Rock in gently and apply knee pressure. Move up and down the lower leg twice, working on Sen Kalathari.

To work on the thigh, fold the recipient's right leg and use your right hand to fix the knee toward the extended left leg. Apply gentle knee pressure up and down the iliotibial band (**fig. 10.4**).

Benefits: Increases circulation and removes waste materials through the venous and lymphatic systems; relieves muscular tension in legs and restless leg syndrome; internally rotates the hip, releasing tension in the lower leg (the tibialis anterior muscle) and along the iliotibial band, which is often tight.

Precautions: Kneeing is especially effective if you have weak wrists or if you are massaging a person who is much larger than you. It is more powerful than palming, however, so be careful not to apply the full weight of your body. Ask for feedback from your recipient and closely monitor his or her comfort level. Never use your knee to massage on the bones. You should feel free to use palming when necessary, such as when working on slender vatas or on people who are much smaller than you.

Vayus activated: Vyana

Ayurvedic tip: This strong variation of sen-line work is most effective for kaphas.

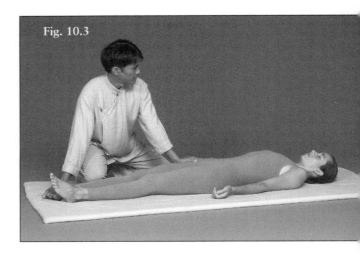

Fig. 10.3

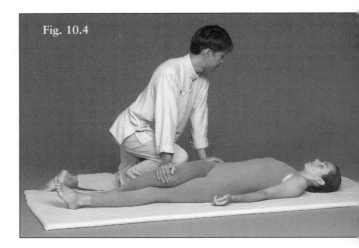

Fig. 10.4

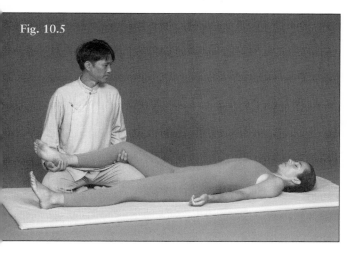

Fig. 10.5

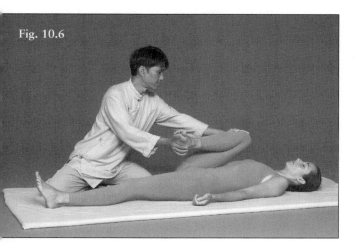

Fig. 10.6

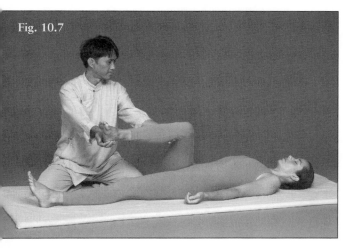

Fig. 10.7

Helicopter V↓↓ P↓ K↓↓↓

Continue sitting in Open Diamond stance beside the recipient's right leg. Place one hand under the recipient's knee and the other under her ankle.

Scoop closer and let the recipient's leg rest on your lap (**fig. 10.5**). Use whirlpool rock to rotate the recipient's knee and hip in a counterclockwise direction (**figs. 10.6 and 10.7**).

For an extended Thai Yoga Massage session, move on to Nataraj. If you're performing a basic Thai Yoga Massage, move on to Demi Lotus.

Benefits: Provides greater range of motion and limbers up the hip joint; relieves tension in the hip and leg; increases mobility of the lumbar spine.

Common mistake: Practitioners do not rock with the whole body.

Precaution: Take care not to lift off of the heels as you perform whirlpool rock, as this can overwork your low back.

Vayus activated: Vyana

Ayurvedic tip: Use gentle and slow pacing for vatas; moderate pacing for pittas; swift and rigorous pacing for kaphas.

† Nataraj V↓↓ P↓↓ K↓↓

Using the momentum of Helicopter, step your right foot forward over the recipient's left leg into an extended Warrior stance. Keeping your right hand on the heel, move your left hand to the knee and instruct the recipient to extend her arms out at shoulder height (**fig. 10.8**). Turning to face the recipient's head, straighten her leg across her midline (**fig. 10.9**).

Place your left hand on the recipient's right thigh and gradually glide her leg down toward your foot. Place your right hand on your right knee and forward rock as you use your left hand to palm up and down the recipient's upper thigh three times, working along Sen Kalathari (**fig. 10.10**).

Benefits: Tones the liver, spleen, and pancreas and is good for digestive health; stretches the abductor muscles; compresses and massages the iliotibial band, an area where many people carry tension.

Vayus activated: Vyana, samana

Ayurvedic tip: Twists are generally tridoshic; be sure to apply the appropriate massage approach for each dosha for maximum effectiveness.

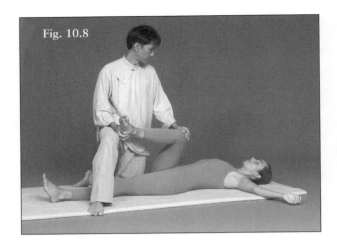

Fig. 10.8

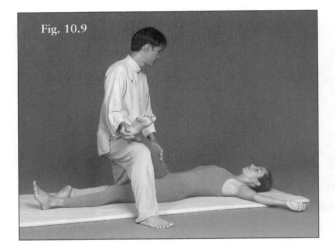

Fig. 10.9

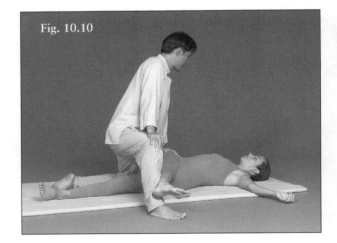

Fig. 10.10

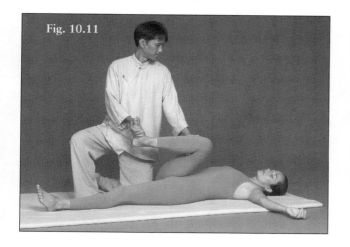

Fig. 10.11

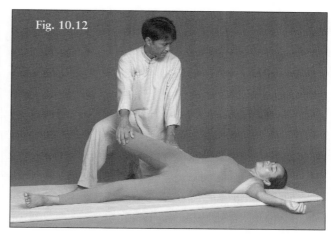

Fig. 10.12

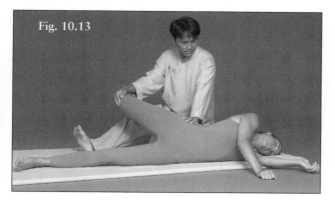

Fig. 10.13

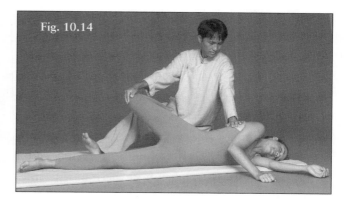

Fig. 10.14

✝ Stringing Bow V↓ P↓↓ K↓↓↓

From Nataraj, maintain an extended Warrior stance as you glide your left knee behind the recipient's lower back. Bring your right hand to the recipient's right instep and your left hand to her right knee. Gently bend the recipient's leg, stepping back into Open Warrior stance alongside her body (**fig. 10.11**).

Move your left hand to the recipient's right hip and gently rotate her right thigh, placing the sole of her right foot on your right hip bone (**fig. 10.12**).

Move your left hand to the recipient's right buttock. Apply gradual pressure with your left hand as you lean back onto your left heel; the motion is as if you are stringing a bow. This creates a supported Locust pose (**fig. 10.13**).

Using your left hand, palm up and down the paravertebral muscles along the right side of the recipient's spine (**fig. 10.14**).

Adaptation: For heavy recipients, bring the leg to rest higher up on your thigh, close to your hip.

Benefits: Extends the hip; relieves low back tension and constipation; massages the internal organs.

Precaution: Apply gradual pressure with a mild stretch for those with lower back pain or sciatica.

Vayus activated: Vyana, udana

Ayurvedic tip: This backbend is great for mobilizing kapha. Go easy with limber vata types—even if they are extremely flexible, a full extension is sometimes not what they need. Do not avoid the posture altogether, just proceed mindfully.

☦ Hugging Tree V P K ▲

From Stringing Bow, come back up into Open Warrior stance on the right side. Interlace your hands underneath the recipient's right knee. Gently swing her knee upward to bring it perpendicular to your hips (**fig. 10.15**).

Come into Kneeling Diamond with your knees supporting the recipient's lower back; wrap both arms around the recipient's right knee (**fig. 10.16**). Gradually sit back in the Diamond stance, allowing the recipient's hips to lift and open (**fig. 10.17**). Maintain a good stretch for three to five breaths.

Benefits: Opens the hip joint; releases tension in the low back; stretches the adductor muscles; relieves sciatica.

Vayus activated: Vyana

Ayurvedic tip: Vatas will especially love this nurturing hug. Hold this cooling posture longer for pittas, as it releases tension in the hips and mid-abdomen.

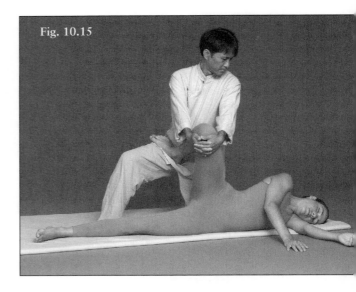

Fig. 10.15

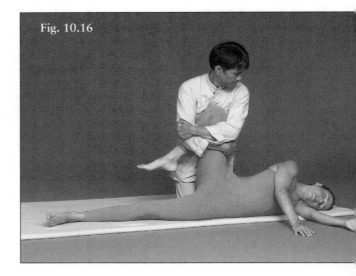

Fig. 10.16

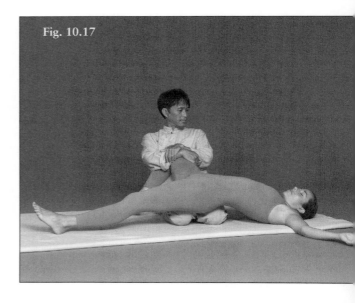

Fig. 10.17

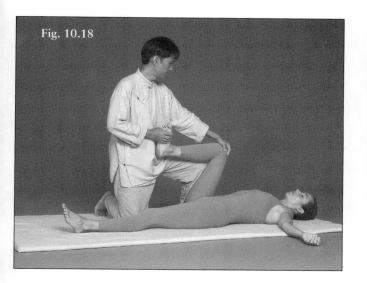

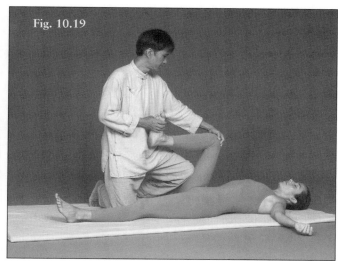

✝ Apana Release V↓↓↓ P↓↓ K↑

From Hugging Tree, place your left palm on the recipient's right knee and your right palm on her right instep. Lift up into Kneeling Diamond, allowing the recipient's hip to return to the mat.

Position your right knee so that it is aligned with the recipient's left (extended) knee. Lift your left leg up into Open Warrior stance. Place your left hand on the recipient's right knee and your right hand on the sole of the foot (**fig. 10.18**).

Fold the recipient's knee toward her chest and place your left knee at the bottom of her hamstring, just above her right knee. Use your left knee to gradually apply the weight of your body to the back of the recipient's thigh (**fig. 10.19**). Work up and down the thigh three times.

Benefits: Relieves constipation and excess gas; tones the internal organs and promotes healthy digestion; compresses and tones the hamstrings.

Precaution: When folding the recipient's knee toward her chest, occasionally she may feel a pinching sensation near the iliac crest, so make sure not to force the movement. If you sense discomfort, gently move on to the next exercise.

Vayus activated: Apana, samana

Ayurvedic tip: In yoga this posture is called Wind-Relieving pose, as it relieves excess apana vayu. It is particularly good for vata types, but you might want to have some incense and a fan nearby!

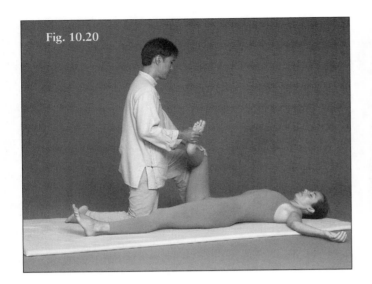

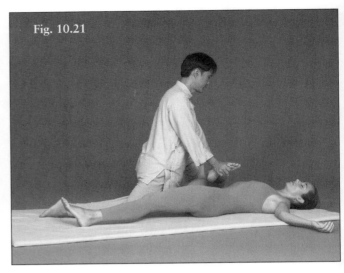

Demi Lotus V↓↓ P↓↓↓ K↓

Lift your left knee into Warrior stance. "Wag" your right leg inward in order to face the recipient's head. Maintain your hand positions and allow the recipient's knee to fall to the side (**fig. 10.20**).

Glide forward in Warrior as you push the sole of the recipient's foot toward her belly. Gradually lean in with your body weight and hold for three to five breaths (**fig. 10.21**).

Benefits: Stretches the iliotibial tract and the hip flexors; compresses and massages the hamstring muscles; improves mobility of the hip.

Common mistake: Practitioner's bent knee exceeds his toes, causing an unsteady stance when pushing forward.

Precautions: Do not twist the knee. Avoid this posture in cases of knee injury or strain, hernia, heart disease, and pregnancy.

Vayus activated: Samana

Ayurvedic tip: This bound posture draws energy inward toward the abdomen and has a cooling effect, making it ideal for pittas.

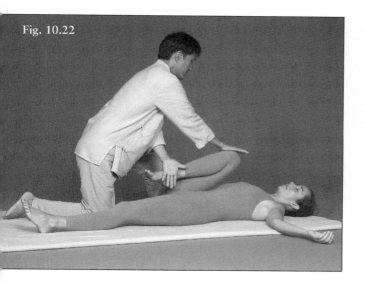

Fig. 10.22

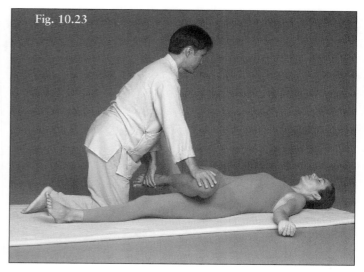

Fig. 10.23

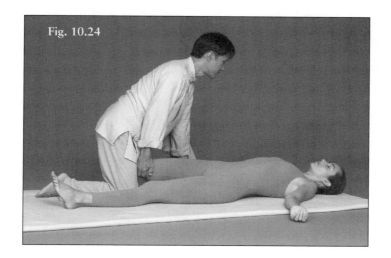

Fig. 10.24

Demi Diamond V↓↓ P↓↓↓ K↓

From Demi Lotus, place your right hand on the recipient's knee and your left hand, palm out, against the recipient's ankle (**fig. 10.22**). Position the recipient's knee across her body and tuck her foot below her buttock, the dorsal side of the foot facing downward (**fig. 10.23**).

Step back into Kneeling Diamond and place the recipient's right kneecap between your thighs (**fig. 10.24**). Squeeze your legs together to create a stable support for the recipient's knee.

Fix your right hand on the recipient's knee. Forward rock as you use your left hand to palm up and down the quadriceps three times (**fig. 10.25**).

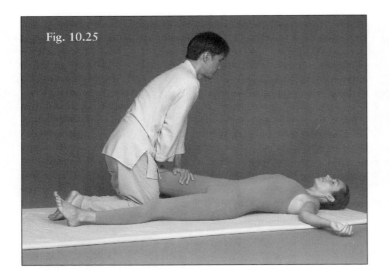

Fig. 10.25

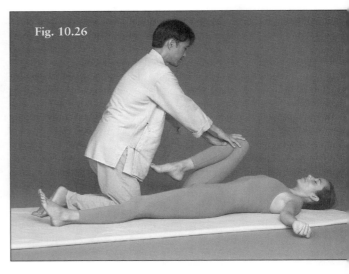

Fig. 10.26

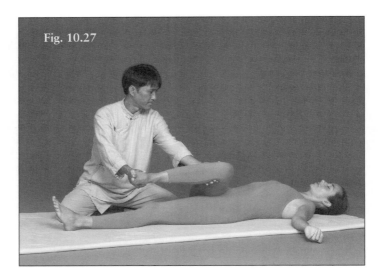

Fig. 10.27

To release, place the recipient's knee in an upright position (**fig. 10.26**). Sit in Open Diamond stance at the recipient's side and apply Helicopter, making clockwise circles, before finally straightening the leg (**fig. 10.27**).

Repeat all of the single-leg postures on the other side before moving on to the back postures.

Benefits: Stretches the quadriceps muscles; tones the abdomen; aids digestion and absorption.

Precautions: Avoid in cases of knee injury or strain, as this can be a very powerful stretch. Move gradually and ask for feedback to assess your recipient's comfort level.

Vayus activated: Samana, apana

Ayurvedic tip: For vatas, use your thighs as a support to avoid lowering the recipient's knee all the way to the mat. For vatas, remember to encourage building strength over flexibility.

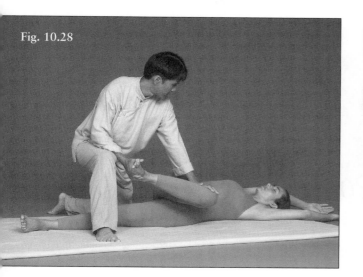

Fig. 10.28

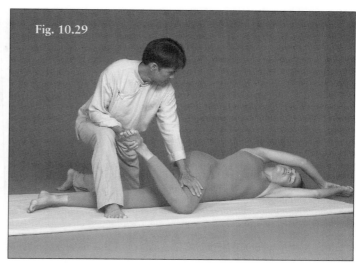

Fig. 10.29

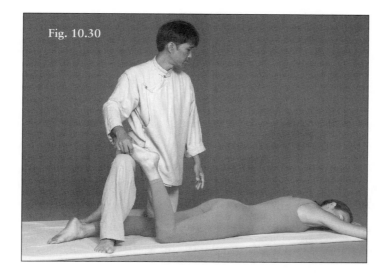

Fig. 10.30

Transitional Flow

In preparation for the back postures, you will now gently flip the recipient to prone using the following technique.

Ask the recipient to raise her arms overhead, extended on the mat. Use whirlpool rock to swing the recipient's knee across the midline as you step into Warrior stance, your front foot over her outside leg (**fig. 10.28**). With the momentum of the whirlpool rock, gently swing the recipient into a prone position (**figs. 10.29 and 10.30**).

Back Postures

In our high-speed, fast-paced culture, aggravated vata is often expressed in the form of back pain and tension. Many individuals go about their daily activities carrying a back full of tense muscles that only massage practitioners can relieve.

According to Ayurveda, the spinal column is the main pathway of energy in the body and the place where unresolved emotions and experiences are stored. By working through tensions in the spine we release energy and allow that energy to flow freely from the coccyx all the way to the crown of the head, the seat of spiritual awareness.

At this point in the Thai Yoga Massage session many recipients will be deeply relaxed; some may even be close to falling asleep. You might want to have towels or small pillows available to tuck under the ankles, upper chest, and lower abdomen, all for the purpose of relaxing the lower back. Placing a pillow under the forehead will keep the nose from being pushed into the floor. When the recipient's head is turned to one side, ask her to periodically move her head to the other side to avoid stiffness in the neck.

For the basic massage you will perform Sole Roll and Janu Pump on each leg before continuing with the remaining back postures. For the extended version, perform the first three exercises on the first leg and then on the second leg before moving on to the remaining back postures. When working on pregnant women, this section of the massage must be modified; from the second trimester on, a pregnant woman should not lie flat on her back for too long. The uterus and the baby are heavy in the abdomen and will compress the vena cava, the main vein at the back of the abdomen, decreasing the return of blood to the heart and thereby decreasing a woman's blood pressure. A decrease in blood pressure will reduce the amount of blood and oxygen going to the baby. Pregnant women often instinctively shift to their side, which provides a more suitable posture for working on their backs. Variations such as Back Pedal or Standing Side Arc offer an excellent alternative for massaging the back in a side-lying posture.

Be careful not to overstretch your pregnant clients and do not perform inverted postures with them. Finally, do not apply pressure to the uterus or marma points.

Sole Roll V↓↓↓ P↓↓ K↓↓

Sit in Open Diamond stance alongside your recipient's lower leg. Lift her left foot to rest on your right thigh (**fig. 11.1**).

Cup the recipient's Achilles tendon with your left hand and roll into her sole with your right forearm (**fig. 11.2**). Gradually work toward the toes, then roll back to the heel.

Switch arms and use your left forearm to roll upward on the recipient's calf (**fig. 11.3**).

Benefits: Compresses the intrinsic muscles of the foot; relieves tension and stiffness in the feet; relieves plantar fasciitis; provides a pressure point massage, toning the lungs.

Vayus activated: Prana

Ayurvedic tip: For bony vata recipients, be sure to create soft support with pillows or cushions. This exercise diffuses pitta irritability and aggression and relieves kapha congestion.

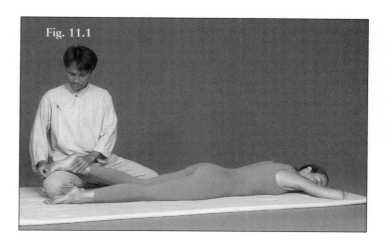
Fig. 11.1

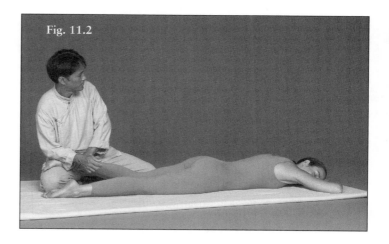
Fig. 11.2

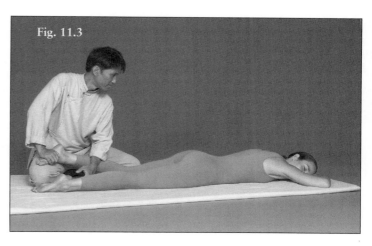
Fig. 11.3

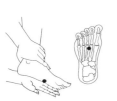

Talahridaya Marma

This marma point is situated at the upper center of the sole in line with the third toe. It is also located at the center of the palm in line with the third finger. Talahridaya marma stimulates the lungs and respiratory system.

Use your elbow to compress the Talahridaya marma for three to five breaths.

Janu Pump V↓ P↓↓↓ K↓

Remain in Open Diamond stance alongside the recipient, aligning the midline of your torso with the recipient's left knee. Hold her left foot with your right hand and place your left fist into the back of the recipient's knee so that your knuckles are facing the recipient's midline (**fig. 11.4**).

Gradually fold the recipient's foot in toward her buttock, applying pressure into the Janu marma point behind the knee (**fig. 11.5**). Hold for three breaths.

Repeat Janu Pump three times. Move with caution, as the back of the knee is a tender area.

For the basic massage, repeat the Sole Roll and Janu Pump on the right leg. For the extended version, include Frog posture on the right side before switching sides. When you've completed Frog posture on the right leg, perform the rest of the back postures bilaterally.

Benefits: Stimulates Janu marma, toning the heart, liver, and spleen; stretches the knee and flexes the hamstring, relieving leg fatigue; increases blood circulation in the legs, flushing away wastes and toxins.

Precautions: Do not apply pressure to Janu marma with the leg extended, as this causes excessive pressure on the knee.

Vayus activated: Samana, prana

Ayurvedic tip: The Janu marma is a major pitta point that releases tension from the heart and liver, both pitta organs. Hold this cooling posture longest for pittas.

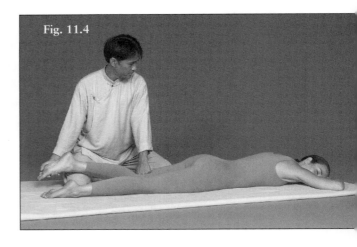

Fig. 11.4

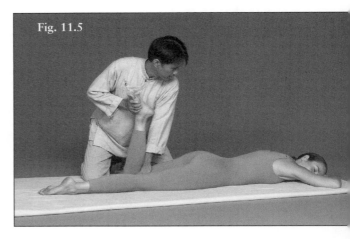

Fig. 11.5

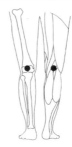

Janu Marma

This marma point has a front and back location; the front point is situated at the root of the knee and the back point is located behind the kneecap.

Applying pressure to Janu marma helps to tone the heart, liver, and spleen. It also lubricates the joints and improves leg circulation.

Janu marma is stimulated during the Janu Pump exercise.

✝ Frog V↓↓↓ P↓↓ K↓

From Janu Pump, lift your left knee into Warrior stance and turn to face the recipient's head. Cup the recipient's left knee with your left hand and the foot with your right hand (**fig. 11.6**). Glide her knee forward to form a 90-degree angle between the foreleg and the thigh (**fig. 11.7**).

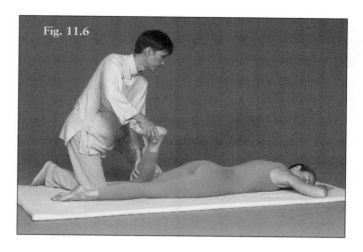

Fig. 11.6

Wag your right leg inward and sit down. Place the blade of your left foot behind the recipient's left knee (**fig. 11.8**). Lift her foot and tuck her toes behind your left knee, interlacing your lower legs together. Now place the ball of your right foot at the back of the recipient's thigh; place your left hand onto the recipient's left calf, and your right hand on her extended leg. Now gently extend your right leg and use the ball of your foot to walk up and down the thigh three to five times (**fig. 11.9**).

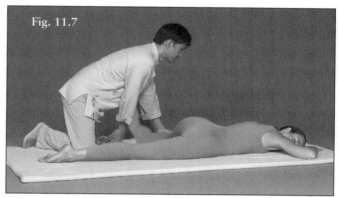

Fig. 11.7

To release, cross your legs and sit up in Kneeling Diamond stance. Extend the recipient's leg into a relaxed position.

Repeat Sole Roll, Janu Pump, and Frog on the right leg.

Benefits: Opens the hip joint and tractions the knee; promotes circulation to the legs; releases tension in the buttocks and lower back; relieves constipation.

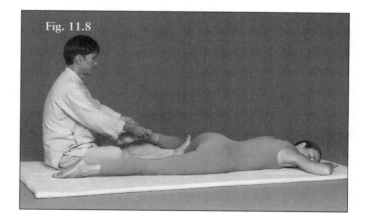

Fig. 11.8

Precaution: When you press in with your heel beware that you do not pinch the skin along the mat. Do not perform this movement on pregnant women or on any recipient who has had hip surgery.

Vayus activated: Vyana, samana

Ayurvedic tip: You can modulate the massage approach here by adjusting your distance from the recipient. Sitting further back from your recipient creates a softer pressure that is best for vatas; sitting closer creates a more intense pressure that benefits pittas and kaphas.

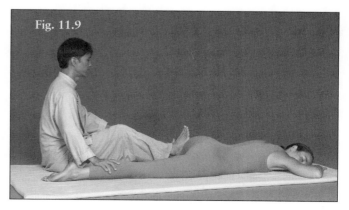

Fig. 11.9

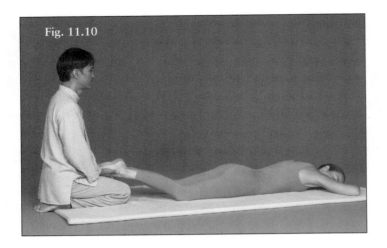

Fig. 11.10

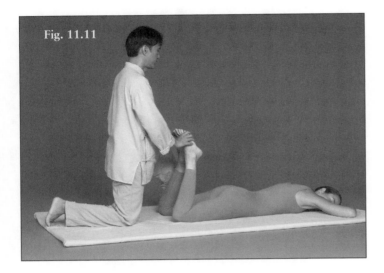

Fig. 11.11

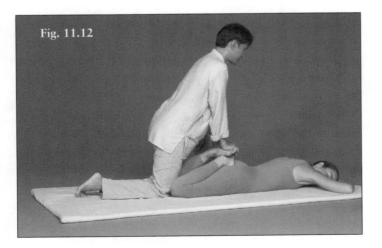

Fig. 11.12

✝ Reverse Lotus V↓↓ P↓↓↓ K↑

Sit in Diamond stance at the recipient's feet so that your thighs are under her feet (**fig. 11.10**).

Lift the recipient's lower legs to a 90-degree angle while you step your left knee up into Warrior stance (**fig. 11.11**).

Cross the recipient's feet and place your hands on them. Glide your Warrior forward, fall in with the full weight of your body, and press the recipient's feet toward her buttocks (**fig. 11.12**). Keep your arms and back straight and hold for three to five breaths. Release back to the 90-degree angle. Repeat two times.

Cross the recipient's feet with the other foot on top and perform Reverse Lotus three times. To release, hold onto the recipient's feet as you knee-walk back and straighten her legs.

Adaptation: Place a pillow between the buttocks and feet if your recipient is very stiff or has knee problems.

Benefits: Increases flexibility of the feet; stretches the hamstrings and iliotibial band.

Precautions: Proceed with extreme care in cases of knee injury or lower back pain.

Vayus activated: Samana, apana

Ayurvedic tip: This bound posture, cooling in its effects, is especially good for pittas. It also helps promote a consistent agni, or digestive fire.

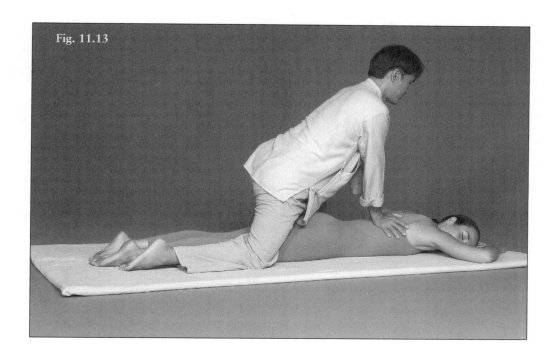

Fig. 11.13

Palming Back V P K ▲

Straddle the recipient in Warrior stance. With arms and back straight, palm up and down the back on either side of the spine (**fig. 11.13**).

Use the full weight of your body to press into the recipient's spinal muscles. Synchronize your breath as you forward rock, encouraging the dance of Thai Yoga Massage to emerge.

Benefits: Works on the paravertebral muscles and autonomic nervous system; relieves back stress and muscle spasms; stimulates the internal organs; aligns the spine.

Precaution: Be careful not to put pressure directly on the spine. Move the recipient's head from side to side every few minutes to prevent stiffness in the neck.

Vayus activated: Vyana, samana

Ayurvedic tip: Follow the appropriate sen-line approach for each dosha. Vatas require a slow and meditative rhythm with an approximate three-second pause before alternating palms; pittas benefit from a cooling and moderate pace with a two-second pause; and kaphas require a more aerobic approach with a one-second pause. For more details on approaches to sen-line work see chapter 6.

Kneeing Back V↑ P↓↓ K↓↓↓

This stronger version of Palming Back can be useful for practitioners with weak or sore wrists. It can also be used in place of palming the back when you want to apply stronger pressure. However, this is a very powerful posture, so you must be gradual in applying your weight to the recipient's back muscles. Never apply more than twenty percent of your full strength.

From Palming Back, position yourself to the left side of the recipient in Kneeling Diamond stance.

Place your left hand on the recipient's left scapula and your right hand on the right side of her sacrum. Lift your right knee and apply gradual pressure to the left buttocks (**fig. 11.14**). Move up along the paravertebral muscles on the left side of the body as far as you are comfortable and stable (**fig. 11.15**).

Move up and down the back three times.

Benefits: Works on the paravertebral muscles and autonomic nervous system; relieves back stress and muscle spasms; stimulates the internal organs; aligns the spine.

Precaution: Ask for feedback from your recipient, closely monitoring her or his comfort level. Never knee directly on the spine. Avoid this posture when working on the elderly.

Vayus activated: Vyana, samana

Ayurvedic tip: This strong sen-line variation is most suitable for kaphas.

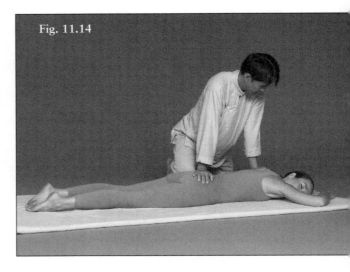
Fig. 11.14

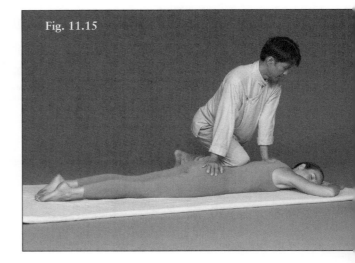
Fig. 11.15

Pillow Cobra V↓↓↓ P↓↓ K↓↓

Place a pillow on the recipient's lower back. Gently sit on the recipient's upper sacrum, your feet flat on the floor (**fig. 11.16**).

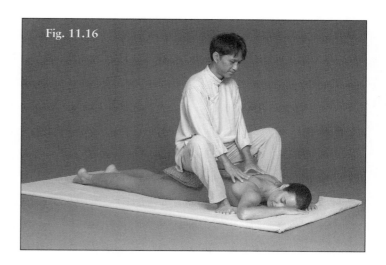

Fig. 11.16

Place the recipient's arms across your thighs, her hands hanging to the side. Grasp the recipient's shoulders from above (**fig. 11.17**).

Using directed breathing, ask the recipient to inhale deeply, then exhale. On the exhale, lean back, leveraging your weight to lift the recipient into a backbend (**fig. 11.18**).

Release by gently returning the recipient's chest to the mat. Ask that the recipient turn her head to the side as the upper body comes back down to the mat.

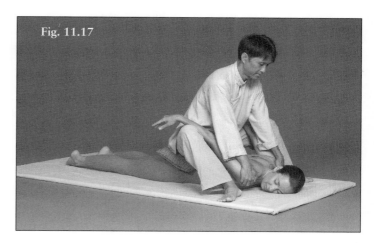

Fig. 11.17

Benefits: Flexes the spine; opens the chest; relieves lower back ache and spinal stiffness; restricts blood flow to the femoral artery, clearing the blood vessels and promoting circulation.

Precaution: Avoid jerky movements.

Common mistake: The practitioner's feet are too close together, causing instability in the posture.

Vayus activated: Prana, vyana, samana

Ayurvedic tip: This is the most stable, easy-to-perform Cobra and is good for all body types.

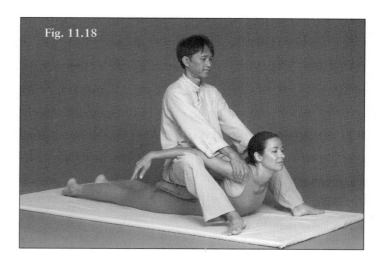

Fig. 11.18

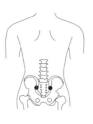

Kukundara Marma

This point is located on either side of the sacrum, just above the fleshy part of the buttocks. Kukundara marma governs blood formation and menstruation.

Kukundara marma is stimulated by Pillow Cobra pose.

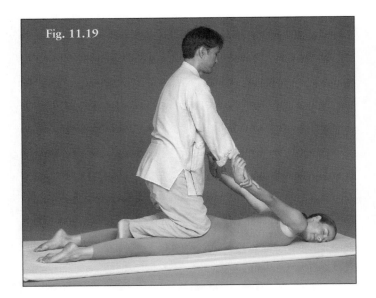

Fig. 11.19

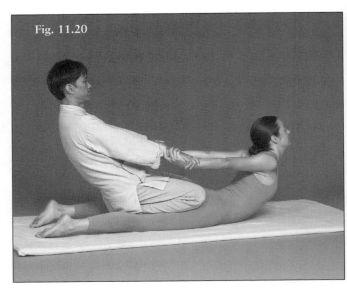

Fig. 11.20

Classical Cobra V↓↓ P↓↓ K↓↓↓

From the sen work on the back move into Kneeling Diamond stance, with your knees fixed on the recipient's buttocks. Ask the recipient to hold onto your wrists or forearms (**fig. 11.19**).

Using directed breathing, ask the recipient to inhale deeply, then exhale. On the exhale lean backward, using the leverage of the movement to gently pull the recipient into a backbend (**fig. 11.20**).

Release by coming back into an upright kneeling position, gently returning the recipient to the mat.

Benefits: Flexes the spine; provides traction through the shoulder girdle, stretching the deltoid muscles; opens the chest; stimulates the internal organs; aids digestion; promotes flexibility of the spine; relieves lower back ache and spinal stiffness; relieves nasal congestion.

Precaution: Avoid performing this posture with recipients who have suffered a dislocated shoulder in the past.

Common mistake: The practitioner's grip of the wrist or forearm is not secure. The knees are not firmly positioned on the buttocks. Be sure to position yourself strongly and securely before performing this posture.

Vayus activated: Vyana, prana, samana

Ayurvedic tip: This chest opener is great for releasing excess kapha. Very fiery pittas can exhale through the mouth or use some of the cooling breathing techniques discussed on page 79 to prevent overheating in this pose.

Transitional Flow

Place the recipient's arms above her head, palms facing down. Come into Warrior stance at the recipient's feet. Grasp the recipient's right foot with your right hand and cup her heel with your left hand (**fig. 11.21**). Extend the right leg, and then gently rotate the recipient toward the medial side to bring her into the supine position (**figs. 11.22 and 11.23**).

This is a fun and effortless way to turn the recipient over. Just remember that most of the rotation occurs at the hip—you will master it in no time! Do not perform this transition on recipients with a history of hip or ankle conditions, such as arthritis, osteoporosis, or replacement joints. Ask those recipients to turn over on their own.

This is the end of the back postures. We're now ready to move on to the double-leg postures.

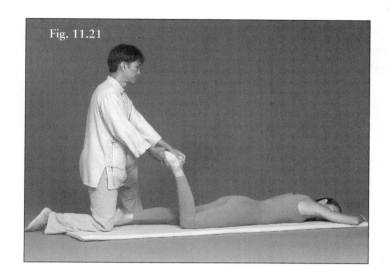

Fig. 11.21

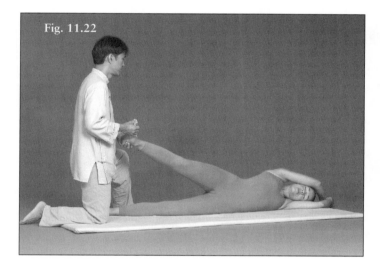

Fig. 11.22

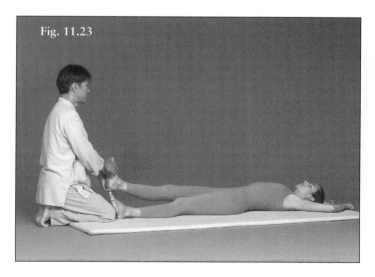

Fig. 11.23

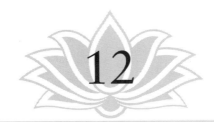

12

Double-Leg Postures

It is especially important to pay attention to body mechanics and alignment while working with the double-leg postures. This is the only portion of the massage in which the practitioner is primarily in a standing position, requiring a certain finesse and mastery over the standing working stances. It is essential to use correct stances to maintain balance and to properly execute the posture, and—most important—to protect your back. Always remember that if you are not aligned or balanced, neither is your recipient.

Pay attention to the duet between you and your recipient, relying on your knowledge of body mechanics to keep your bodies in good alignment, and use common sense! This is particularly important when applying the Ayurvedic approach for each client. If you are a petite vata person it may be difficult to apply the strong pressure and dynamic pace recommended for your large-framed or heavy kapha clients. In these cases it is always better to preserve your own well-being and save the recommended massage approach for the less demanding portions of the massage.

Since many of these postures involve placing the recipient in inversions, they should be performed with a clear understanding of contraindications. Never perform inversions on recipients with high blood pressure or cervical spine problems, as these conditions tend to be aggravated by inverted movements. Inversions are also unsuitable during pregnancy, menstruation, or if your client has arteriosclerosis, a thickening of the artery walls that leads to impaired blood circulation.

† Crescent Moon V↓↓ P↓↓↓ K↓↓

Sit in Open Diamond stance at your recipient's feet. Ask the recipient to place her hands at her sides. Grasp the recipient's left foot and cross it over her right ankle (**fig. 12.1**). Glide her legs to the her left, allowing the feet to hang over the edge of the mat (**fig. 12.2**).

Step into Warrior stance and pick up the recipient's right hand. Gradually lift up into Tai Chi stance, gently applying traction to the arm (**fig. 12.3**). Walk in a semicircle until you are standing above the recipient's head.

Sit down behind the recipient and place your left foot on her left shoulder. Maintain gentle pressure on the shoulder while you fall back with your body weight and stretch the extended arm (**fig. 12.4**).

Hold for three to five breaths. Repeat the stretch two times.

Proceed with Tea Pot before changing sides.

Benefits: Stretches the serratus anterior, transverse abdominus, and quadratus lumborum; opens the hip abductors.

Precaution: Take care not to put your foot on the recipient's hair or face.

Vayus activated: Vyana

Ayurvedic tip: This cooling elongation is good for diffusing excess pitta energy.

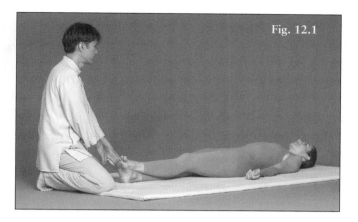
Fig. 12.1

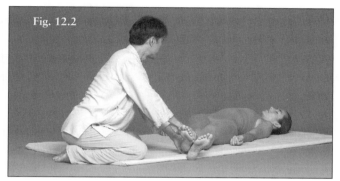
Fig. 12.2

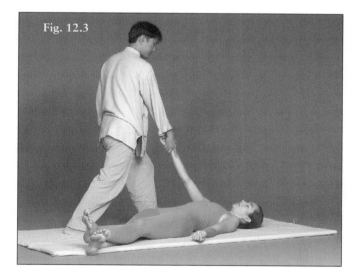
Fig. 12.3

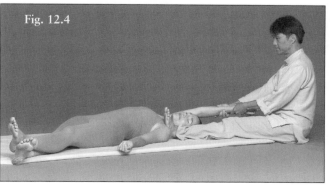
Fig. 12.4

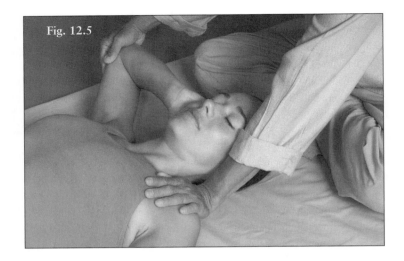

Fig. 12.5

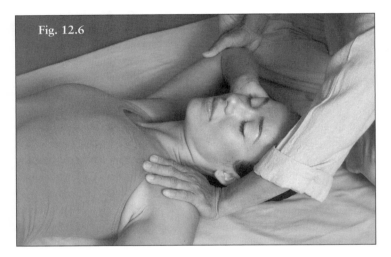

Fig. 12.6

✝ Tea Pot V↓↓ P↓↓ K↓↓↓

From Crescent Moon, come to a seated cross-legged position. Bend the recipient's right arm and cup her hand over her ear (**fig. 12.5**).

With your right hand on the recipient's right elbow and your left hand on her shoulder, gently glide her head to the left. Lightly pull her elbow toward your center, providing a good neck and side stretch (**fig. 12.6**).

To release, gently bring the recipient's head back to center and place her arm alongside the body. Repeat Crescent Moon and Tea Pot on the opposite side.

Benefits: Stretches the triceps; flexes the cervical spine laterally.

Precaution: Proceed gently and avoid all jerky movements.

Vayus activated: Udana, prana

Ayurvedic tip: As you practice this posture imagine that you are pouring an abundance of prana into the head, energizing the mind and senses. This posture is great for kaphas!

Tortoise V↓↓ P↓↓ K↓↓↓

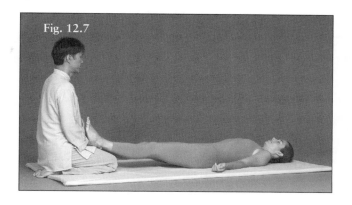

Fig. 12.7

Move to the recipient's feet and come into Diamond stance. Return the recipient's legs to center and place her feet on your thighs (**fig. 12.7**).

Cup the recipient's heels and, in one fluid motion, push her legs upward as you lift up into Warrior stance (**fig. 12.8**). The palms of your hands remain on the recipient's heels. Keep your arms and back straight.

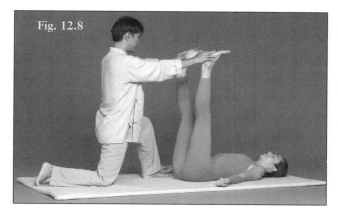

Fig. 12.8

Curl the toes of your right foot and lift yourself into a standing position. Separate the recipient's legs and step forward into Horse Riding stance, bending the recipient's legs, allowing her knees to fall to the side with respect to her flexibility. Walk in close so that your knees are pressed into the back of the recipient's thighs close to her buttocks. Rock forward while pressing on her heels (**fig. 12.9**).

When performing the extended massage, continue with Hip Swirl. For the basic massage, to release this position hold onto the recipient's heels while you walk back and extend her legs. Continue with Thai Lute.

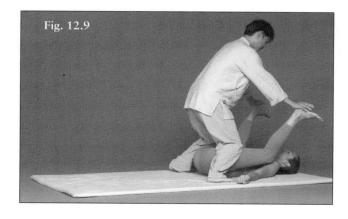

Fig. 12.9

Adaptations: When working on flexible clients, knee up and down the gluteus maximus and hamstrings three times. When working on heavy clients or clients with large frames, move to the side and work on one leg at a time (**fig. 12.10**).

Benefits: Tones the buttocks and elongates the spine; relieves constipation.

Precautions: Maintain a steady and firm posture. Avoid slipping off balance—do not knee beyond your comfortable reach.

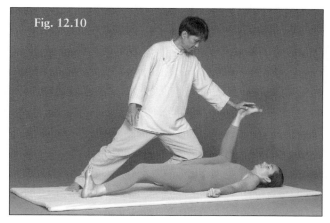

Fig. 12.10

Vayus activated: Udana, samana

Ayurvedic tip: Tortoises are slow and peaceful, making them quite kaphic in nature. Here you are placing the tortoise on its back to open and release stagnant kapha energy.

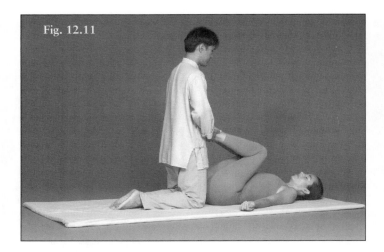

Fig. 12.11

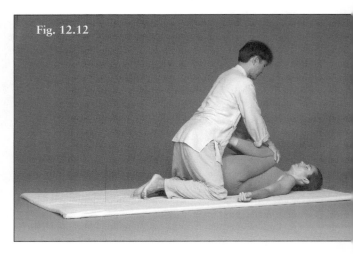

Fig. 12.12

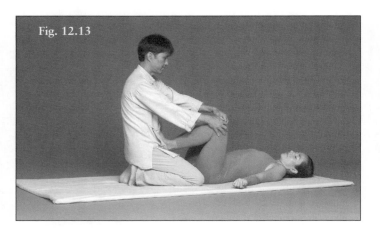

Fig. 12.13

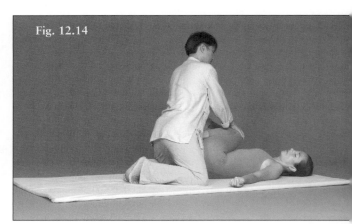

Fig. 12.14

† Hip Swirl V↓↓↓ P↓↓↓ K↓

From Tortoise pose, hold onto the recipient's heels and lower yourself into Kneeling Diamond stance, two inches behind the recipient's buttocks (fig. 12.11).

Place the recipient's feet onto your abdomen and support yourself by placing your hands on her knees (fig. 12.12). Lean forward with the weight of your body and use whirlpool rock to roll the recipient's legs and hips (figs. 12.13 and 12.14). Complete five rotations, then repeat the circles in the opposite direction.

To release, push the recipient's knees forward, rise up into Kneeling Diamond stance, and grasp the heels. Knee-walk back to extend her legs.

Benefits: Opens the hip joints; releases tension in the lower back and sacroiliac joints.

Vayus activated: Samana, vyana

Ayurvedic tip: Imagine that you are swirling energy inward to the core of the abdomen, igniting the digestive fire of agni.

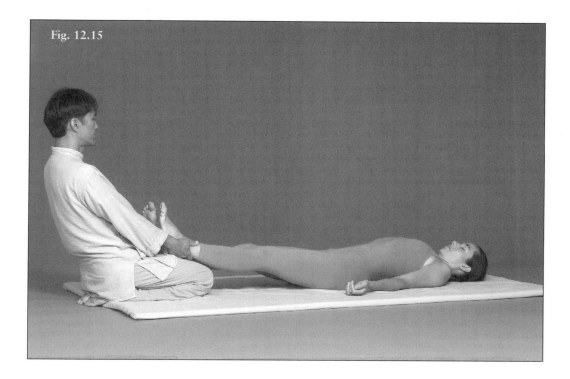

Fig. 12.15

Thai Lute V↓↓ P↓↓↓ K↓

Sit in Open Diamond stance at the recipient's feet. Place the recipient's heels on your thighs. Grasp the heels and lean back with the weight of your body (**fig. 12.15**). Maintain this elongated traction for three to five breaths. Repeat three times.

To release, gently lower the recipient's feet to the mat. As a possible modification, bring the legs together and support the heels with one hand while moving into Warrior stance. With your free hand, place a pillow under the recipient's knees and then gently lower her legs to the mat. This will lift the recipient's knees, relaxing her spine in preparation for the abdominal massage.

Benefits: Aligns the spine; releases tension in the lower spine, sacrum, and abdomen; relieves sciatica; provides a cooling counterposture to Tortoise.

Precautions: Be careful not to pinch the feet.

Vayus activated: Apana, samana

Ayurvedic tip: This cooling posture is particularly good for fiery pittas.

Transitional Flow

Sit in Diamond stance to the left of the recipient.

This is the end of the double-leg postures. We are now ready to move on to the abdomen, chest, arm, and hand postures.

13

Postures for the Abdomen, Chest, Arms, and Hands

In the West we often initiate a conversation by commenting on the weather or asking "How are you?" In contrast, initial greetings in the East frequently revolve around the topic of food or digestion. For example, a common Chinese welcome translates as "Have you eaten today?" In some areas of India a burp after the meal is actually considered to be a compliment to the chef! Such an awareness of nutrition and acceptance of metabolic processes arises from the Ayurvedic belief that digestion is the key to all health and longevity.

During this portion of the session we massage the abdomen and appropriate marma points, thereby tonifying the digestive organs and igniting the digestive fire of agni. As discussed in chapter 3, each dosha has a site of accumulation along the digestive tract; it is the stomach for kapha, the small intestines for pitta, and the colon for vata.

Each of our vital organs is also governed by one of the three constitutions, and imbalances in one dosha may be expressed by imbalances in a particular organ. In order to promote the removal of wastes and toxins, you may spend more time massaging those organs related to your recipient's predominant dosha (see page 31). Remember to apply a natural and intuitive approach while integrating these details, to avoid disrupting the rhythmic flow of the Thai Yoga Massage session.

The abdomen contains most of our major internal organs; for that reason it can be a very sensitive part of the body to massage. Some people can be shy about being touched in this area, so first ask your recipient if he or she would like to be massaged on the abdomen before you actually begin. Do not massage or touch the breasts.

Avoid massaging the abdomen if the recipient has an intense stomachache. Instead, a longer massage on the back, on the side, or in the sitting position is recommended. Avoid abdominal massage on pregnant women. If the recipient feels tension in the low back, place a pillow under the knees; this relaxes a tight low back and reduces pressure on the ovaries for women.

Begin the abdomen exercises with the techniques of Lay-a-Brick and Sun-Moon Stroke to calm and soothe the client. Follow the recipient's breath and calmly synchronize your movement to this flow. When you feel the recipient is relaxed, lightly apply pressure on the five organ-reflex points.

Lay-a-Brick V P K ▲

This technique was passed on to me by my mother, who would place a brick on my abdomen to calm my hyperactive disposition. Although my mother was not aware of the exact terminology, she was working on a primary energy point known in Ayurveda as the Basti marma.

Sit in Diamond stance alongside the recipient. Place your right hand over the area just below the recipient's belly button and synchronize your breath with hers (**fig. 13.1**).

With a straight arm, rock in gently with the weight of your body on an exhalation and ease off on the inhalation.

Benefits: Encourages deep breathing and has a calming effect on the entire body. Stimulates Basti marma, which helps to regulate the urinary and reproductive organs.

Vayus activated: Samana, apana

Ayurvedic tip: Lay-a-Brick is probably the most natural sedative that can be prescribed for our anxious and hyperactive vata recipients. Almost everyone can benefit from this exercise, particularly in our current vata-dominated culture.

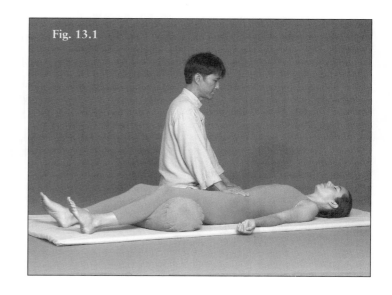

Fig. 13.1

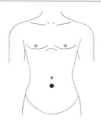

Basti Marma

This urinary point is located between the pubic symphysis and belly button. Basti marma is a large point, approximately four finger-widths in diameter. Working on this point detoxifies the urinary tract and encourages deep yogic breathing, producing a calming effect.

Basti marma is naturally stimulated during the Lay-a-Brick exercise.

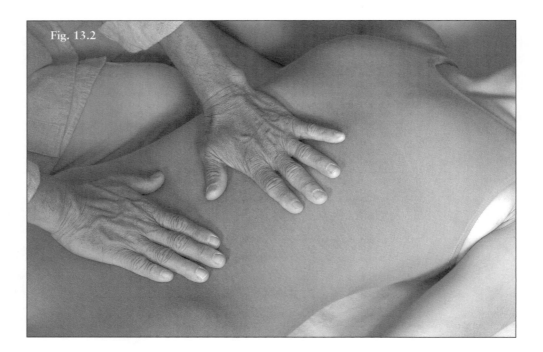

Fig. 13.2

Sun-Moon Stroke V P K ▲

Continuing to sit in Diamond stance alongside the recipient, circle one hand in a clockwise manner around the perimeter of the abdomen, following the path of the large intestine (**fig. 13.2**). This represents the sun. The other hand follows, making the same rotation, but lifts off the abdomen when it comes into contact with the sun hand. This half-circle stroke represents the moon. This stroke creates a soothing effect in preparation for palming.

Benefits: Prepares the recipient for palming techniques; circulates healing energy throughout the internal organs and helps to relax the body.

Vayus activated: Samana, apana

Ayurvedic tip: In Ayurveda, proper digestion is the key to all health. Here, the clockwise stroking moves in the direction of the digestive process, thus promoting absorption and elimination.

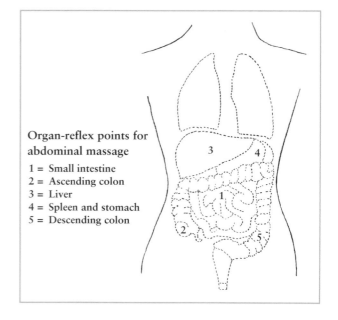

Organ-reflex points for abdominal massage

1 = Small intestine
2 = Ascending colon
3 = Liver
4 = Spleen and stomach
5 = Descending colon

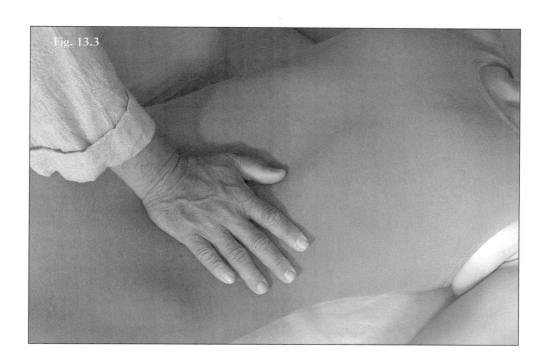

Fig. 13.3

Massaging the Organ-Reflex Points V P K ▲

Palming

Sit in Diamond stance alongside the recipient with your palm on organ-reflex point 1. Wait for an exhalation to rock in gently with the weight of your body (**fig. 13.3**). Hold for one full inhale and exhale, then ease off with the next inhalation.

Repeat on points 2 through 5.

The Doshas and their Corresponding Organ Points

Vata: points 2 (ascending colon) and 5 (descending colon)

Pitta: points 1 (small intestine) and 3 (liver)

Kapha: point 4 (stomach)

For a more detailed discussion of the relationship between the doshas and the organs, see "Areas of Accumulation" on page 29.

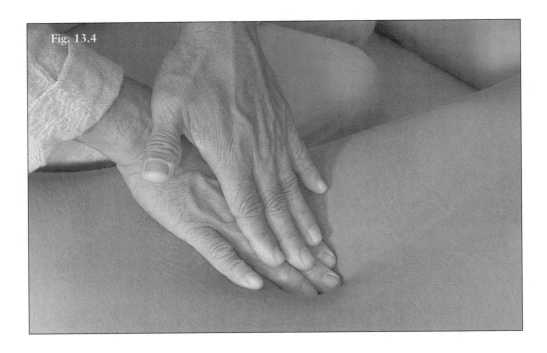

Fig. 13.4

Finger Pressing

From Diamond stance, place the fingers of both hands on organ-reflex point 1 (**fig. 13.4**). Wait for an exhalation to rock in gently with the weight of your body. Don't push in sharply with your fingertips; simply ease in with your fingers and ease off with the inhalation.

Repeat on points 2 through 5.

Repeat the Sun-Moon Stroke to end this part of the session.

Benefits: Releases tension in the belly; helps to relieve constipation, as working in the clockwise direction assists with elimination; stimulates the digestive fire of agni.

Precaution: Do not press strongly on recipients with heart disease. Do not perform these abdominal massages on pregnant women.

Vayus activated: Samana, apana

Ayurvedic tip: You can spend more time on the points corresponding to the organs of accumula-

tion that relate to each recipient's predominant dosha. Add one more palming for each appropriate point.

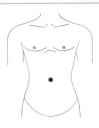

Nabhi Marma

This marma point is centered at the belly button and expands out into a circle approximately four finger-widths in diameter. Nabhi marma is the main point for the digestive system and is a major pitta point. It controls the small intestines and the digestive fire of agni. Nabhi marma corresponds to organ-reflex point 1 and is stimulated during the abdominal massage.

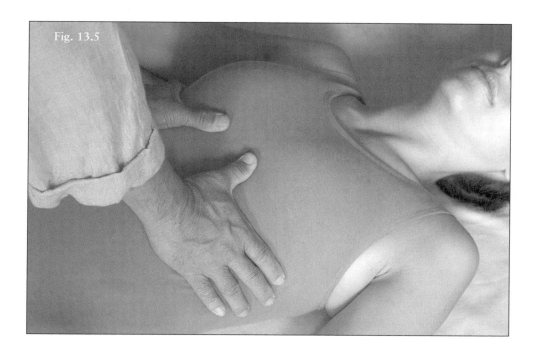

Fig. 13.5

Opening the Chest V↓↓ P↓↓ K↓↓↓

Position yourself in Warrior stance beside the recipient. Place your hands on the ribs, the heels of the hands facing the middle of the chest (**fig. 13.5**). The fingers follow the ribs along the side of the rib cage.

On an exhalation, fall in with the weight of your body, spreading the chest. Ease off on the next inhalation. Move slightly upward on the rib cage and repeat.

Now do the same movement beginning just above the floating ribs.

Move to the upper chest and apply a third time just below the shoulders.

Benefits: Expands the chest and compresses the costal cartilage, maintaining flexibility through the rib cage; relieves chest tension; aligns and elongates the thoracic spine.

Precaution: Spread your weight evenly through your palms. Avoid pressing on the breasts. Do not perform this posture on recipients with osteoporosis.

Vayus activated: Prana, udana

Ayurvedic tip: This chest-opening posture breaks up excess phlegm, making it ideal for kaphas. This exercise benefits all three doshas, especially during the high-kapha seasons of late winter and early spring.

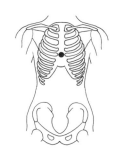

Hridaya Marma

This point is located at the center of the sternum. It controls the fourth chakra (Anahata, the heart chakra), governs the circulatory system, and boosts immunity.

Place the pad of your three middle fingers at the center of the sternum. Apply gentle circular pressure for three to five breaths.

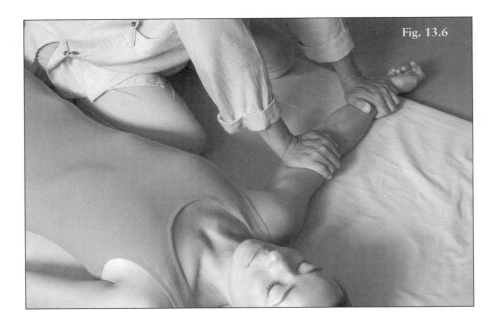

Fig. 13.6

Palming Arms V P K ▲

Sit on the recipient's right side in Open Diamond stance. Bring the recipient's arm to a 90-degree angle.

Place your left hand on the recipient's wrist and your right hand above the crook of the elbow. Using bamboo rocking, palm up and down the recipient's arm (**fig. 13.6**). One hand moves from the wrist to the elbow and the other moves from the elbow to just below the underarm.

Proceed to the hand massage on this side before switching arms.

Benefits: Tones the brachial, ulnar, and radial arteries; compresses along the intraosseous sheath in the forearm; clears lactic acid and relieves fatigue and numbness in the arms.

Precaution: Take care to palm along the center of the arm using moderate pressure, as this can be a very powerful posture.

Vayus activated: Vyana

Ayurvedic tip: Follow the appropriate sen-line approach for each dosha. Vatas require a slow and meditative rhythm, with an approximate three-second pause before alternating palms; pittas benefit from a cooling and moderate pace with a two-second pause; kaphas require a more aerobic approach with a one-second pause. For more details on sen-line work see chapter 6.

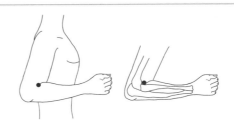

Kurpara Marma

This point is located at the elbow joint and is about three finger-widths in diameter. Kurpara marma controls the liver, spleen, blood, and circulatory system.

Use the thumb and apply gradual and gentle pressure to Kurpara marma for three to five breaths.

Hand Massage V P K ▲

Remain in Open Diamond stance alongside the recipient. Place one hand on the recipient's palm and the other hand below the underarm.

Rock forward into the palm of the recipient's hand (**fig. 13.7**). Change position as needed to palpate the recipient's entire palm.

Turn the recipient's hand around and palm the back of the hand in the same manner.

Sit back into a cross-legged position and bring the recipient's hand with you to work on the Kshipra marma (**fig. 13.8**). Finally, using bamboo rock, squeeze the hand from side to side in a rhythmic, pendulum-like motion (**fig. 13.9**).

Change arms and repeat Palming Arms and the Hand Massage on the other side before closing the session with the Marma Face Massage.

Benefits: Promotes circulation and cleansing of the heart; releases endorphins; relieves carpal tunnel syndrome.

Vayus activated: Vyana, prana

Ayurvedic tip: By working on the Kshipra marma we are cleansing the heart and blood, providing a pitta detox.

Transitional Flow

Sit comfortably in a cross-legged position a few inches behind the recipient's head in preparation for the face massage. We're now ready to move on to the session's close.

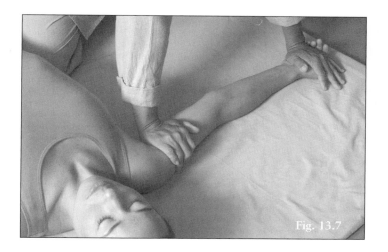
Fig. 13.7

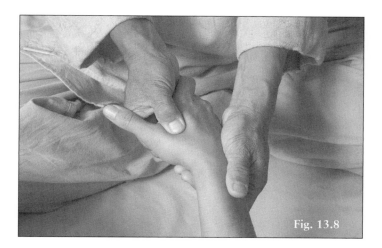
Fig. 13.8

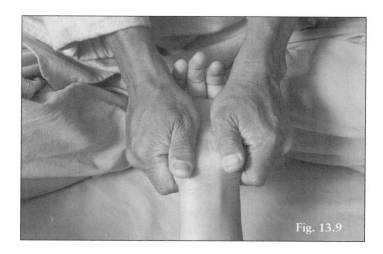
Fig. 13.9

14

Session Closure

We conclude a Thai Yoga Massage session much like a yoga class—with the recipient lying on her back in Savasana. Now that the recipient is completely relaxed and full of renewed prana there is one last and much-loved movement to perform—a face massage! The facial techniques of a traditional Thai massage are chopping, squeezing, pinching, and slapping; however, ending a session this way shocks the body (and the mind) of most Western recipients. This is not a very relaxed way to end a massage.

Our approach to the session closure provides an alternative to the abrupt method commonly used in Thailand. We finish with a gentle rubbing and stroking of the facial muscles. By stimulating the nerves that govern the facial muscles we improve the tone of those muscles and prevent wrinkles, providing a natural face-lift.

Keeping with the tradition of working the marma points, we include light circulation of pressure points with the fingers. As you work on the facial points, visualize each one as an essential transfer station that passes vital energy to the sensory organs, nasal cavity, and brain. Encourage a free and peaceful flow of energy through each marma point.

When beginning the massage, move in slowly and gently with your hands so as not to startle the recipient. At the end, remove your hands slowly and gently. Before beginning the facial massage you may place a few drops of essential oil on your wrists to provide basic aromatherapy according to your client's predominant dosha. (For a list of essential oils that correspond to each dosha, please refer to page 27.)

Following the face massage, finish the session as you began: with a moment of silence in Namaskar.

Marma Face Massage V P K ▲

Sit close to the recipient's head. Stroke the side of the recipient's face in a soft and nurturing way (**fig. 14.1**). Press gently at the temples to stimulate the Shanka marma and relieve any lingering tension at the head (**fig. 14.2**). Massage the ears, home to many acupressure points. Rub and squeeze the entire ear, giving special attention to the earlobes. Recipients generally love this! Finish by stroking the side of the recipient's face again in preparation for the marma face massage.

Now begin to work the marma points by applying circular thumb pressure to stimulate all the facial marma points shown below. The only point that may be difficult to reach with the thumbs is the Vidhura point, below the ear, in which case you may use the index and middle fingers. Gently rub each point for approximately three to five breaths for a general massage.

Benefits: Provides a natural Ayurvedic face-lift; increases the flow of prana to the head, clearing the senses and mind.

Vayus activated: Prana, udana

Ayurvedic tip: Apply a few drops of essential oil on your wrist for Ayurvedic aromatherapy. For example, patchouli is good for vata, sandalwood benefits pitta, and eucalyptus is a good scent for kapha.

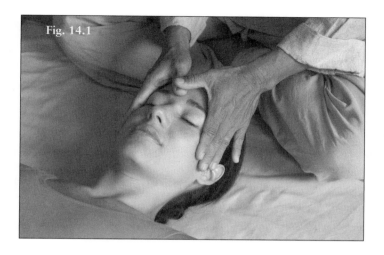

Fig. 14.1

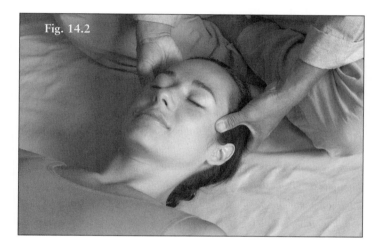

Fig. 14.2

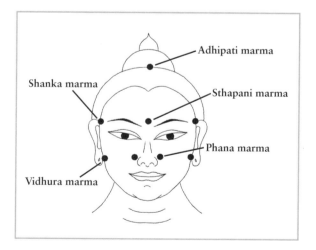

Namaskar V P K ▲

Now that you are at the end of your session with the recipient, it is important to have a formal approach for departure. This is particularly true when you embody Ayurvedic qualities that counterbalance your recipient. If we do not make a proper closure, our own doshic constitution may be influenced by our work.

In order to initiate this closure, sit behind the recipient, your hands together at your heart in the Namaskar prayer posture. Take a moment to empty your thoughts; be mindful of your breath and detach from the doshic approach you embodied. You may also use a pleasant-sounding bell or a soothing *Om* chant to return to a neutral state.

This moment of silence allows you to detach from the doshic quality embodied during the massage and center yourself according to your own doshic makeup. It also provides a quiet moment to reconnect with the true purpose of Ayurveda and Thai Yoga Therapy, to plant the seeds of loving-kindness and to cultivate metta in all that we do.

PART 4

❖❖

A Thai Yoga Therapy Wellness Program

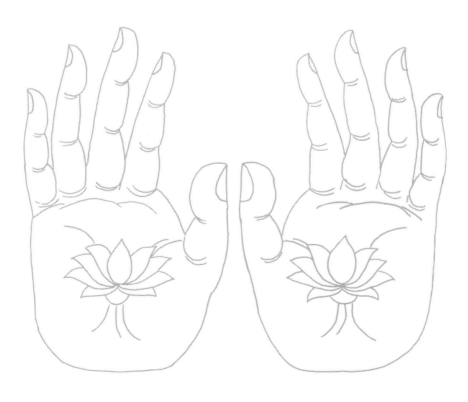

15

Yoga Approaches for the Three Doshas

Once you establish rapport with your clients, it is possible to expand the wisdom of Ayurveda into other aspects of daily living. Every day we are faced with choices that affect our overall sense of harmony—from what we eat to how we exercise and how we spend our leisure time. Many individuals feel wonderful just after a massage or yoga session, but they quickly lose this equilibrium due to poor nutritional choices, lack of appropriate exercise, or a hectic lifestyle.

The beauty of Ayurveda is that it provides a scientific approach that teaches us how to make daily choices to increase peace and maintain sustained wellness for ourselves and clients. The key to understanding how to navigate our way through these daily decisions is to know who we are—which, according to Ayurveda, means understanding our doshic constitution. With this knowledge we can build a lifestyle that complements our doshic body type, bringing Ayurveda into our lives for the duration of our lives.

The wellness program introduced in this section is comprised of three components—yoga postures for home practice, nutritional recommendations, and lifestyle tips. Providing simple and clear recommendations to our clients in these areas will support their overall health and well-being, as well as establish a stronger therapeutic rapport.

YOGA APPROACH FOR VATAS

Individuals of a predominantly vata nature benefit from a yoga practice that is slow, gentle, and meditative in approach. The primary focus of the practice should be on establishing balance and core strength rather than developing flexibility. Although flexibility often comes naturally for the slender and wiry vata body type, individuals of this nature should avoid overflexing or overextending the body. Overstretching can have an adverse effect and may stimulate the sympathetic nervous system, the aspect of the nervous system that prepares the body for action.

Vata postures should aim to tone the parasympathetic nervous system, which produces a calming effect on the body and mind—something most vatas need. Yoga postures should therefore be selected for their ability to build strength, stability, and steadiness. Gentle yoga classes that include plenty of time for deep breathing and relaxation are preferable to those that cause exertion or pain.

Vata Yoga Series

The yoga exercises that balance and restore vata include motionless balancing postures, such as forward bends, and standing balancing poses; sitting postures and seated spinal twists also help to slow down and ground vata. Mild backbends are good, in moderation, as they help to relieve vata stiffness and tension in the sacrum and along the spine. Mild inversions can be helpful for nourishing the upper extremities and brain, but they can cause exertion or fatigue if done in excess.

Vata individuals should take care to avoid abrupt movements, jumping, or significant sweating during a session—leave that to the kaphas! Rather, vatas should focus on maintaining even and consistent energy throughout the duration of a yoga session. Yoga postures should be held long enough to slow the mind and promote deep breathing, but they should never cause exertion or pain. Vatas should also make sure to practice all exercises evenly on both sides of the body to instill regularity and balance, qualities often lacking in their practice and lifestyle.

As discussed in chapter 3, each dosha is associated with a region of the body in which tensions accumulate; these areas of accumulation therefore may require special attention during a yoga session. The organs and regions of the body where vata types tend to be sensitive include the colon (large intestine), spine, back muscles, pelvis, thighs, kidneys, ears, bones, and hollow and dry cavities of the body.

Every yoga session personalized for a vata constitution should be completed with a generous period of relaxation in Savasana, with the practitioner lying on the back and breathing deeply into the abdomen. Vata individuals will need at least fifteen minutes of relaxation for a ninety-minute yoga session. Pillows, blankets, eye pillows, and any props that help to comfort and warm the vata individual are recommended.

YOGA FOR VATAS

 VATA DOSHA

Approach to practice	Slow, meditative, warming, gentle, strengthening and balancing
Vayus to awaken	Prana, apana, vyana, samana
Recommended postures	The best postures for vatas promote stillness, balance, and stability, with long periods of relaxation.
	Forward bends: Offer relief for excessive vata, producing calm and stillness; excellent for releasing vata in the back, where stiffness and tension tends to accumulate; for vatas, forward bends are best combined with gentle backbends
	Backward bends: Excellent for reducing vata, if done gently and slowly; small backbends such as Cobra and Locust help to relieve vata kyphosis and curvature of the shoulder
	Spinal twists: Excellent for vatas, as they help to relieve nervous tension and tonify the colon
	Mild inversions: Benefit vatas when done in moderation; help to promote circulation and nourish the blood and brain
	Sitting postures: Help to ground vata, particularly if held for a long time
	Standing postures: Simple standing postures or standing balancing poses are best for vatas, as they promote the downward, grounding movement of apana vayu
	Avoid overexertion that may cause fatigue or pain.
Holds	Long, easy holds with repetition; avoid moving or fidgeting during holds
Areas of concentration	Vata's site of accumulation: Colon (large intestine)
	Other key vata areas: Spine, back muscles, pelvis, thighs, kidneys, ears, bones, hollow and dry cavities of the body
Disease tendency	Nervous system disorders, pain, arthritis, mental disorders, constipation

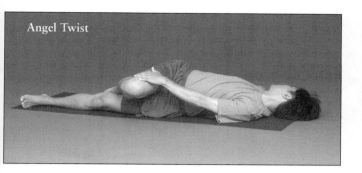

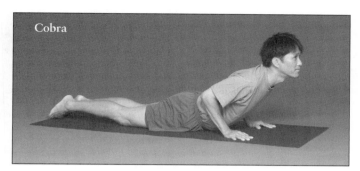

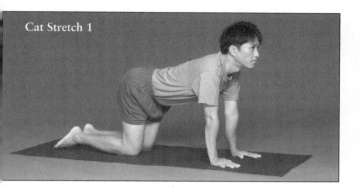

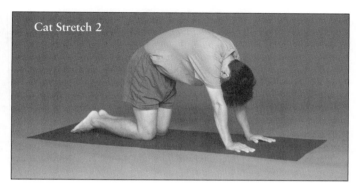

Yoga postures for vatas emphasize balance, gentle stretches, nurturing poses,
and long periods of relaxation.

Vayus for the Vata Constitution

As we mentioned in chapter 3, an understanding of the five directions of prana, the vayus, is a powerful tool for balancing one's doshic type. A well-balanced yoga program will attend to all five vayus. Yet there are particular vayus that are specifically good for each doshic type. Sometimes simply being aware of the direction of the vayus can help to calm, increase, or channel energy to specific areas of weakness or low energy within the body.

Although vata individuals actually benefit from awakening a subtle combination of most of the vayus, the best vayus for these individuals are the inward movement of prana and the downward movement of apana. The one exception is the upward movement of udana vayu, which in excess can destabilize and imbalance vata.

A vata yoga series should include a generous proportion of forward bends, which recharge the pranic battery and have a revitalizing effect on the body. Pranayama breathing exercises, such as Anuloma Viloma, help to renew and balance vata energy, which is often erratic or low. The downward movement of apana helps to ground vata and is activated by mild spinal twists, standing postures, and relaxation poses.

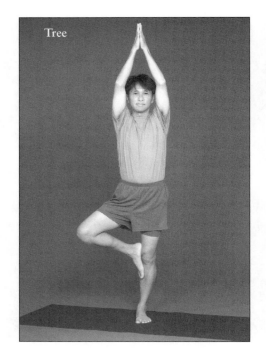

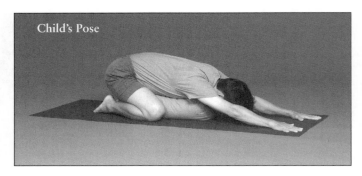

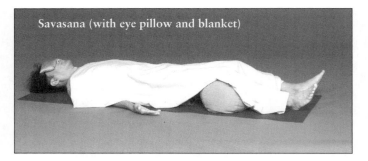

More yoga postures for vatas

YOGA APPROACH FOR PITTAS

The fiery pitta is best suited to a cooling, soft, relaxing approach to yoga that diffuses excessive heat or irritability in the body. Postures should be nonvigorous, have a cooling effect on the head and blood, and aim at calming the heart.

Pitta individuals have the drive and willpower to excel in a yoga practice, which can result in a tendency toward becoming overly competitive and serious in the practice. Individuals of this nature will benefit from a noncompetitive atmosphere that allows them to let go of control and effort. Moderate hatha yoga classes that focus on alignment would be preferable to the more aerobic forms of yoga performed in a heated room or those that cause excessive sweating. The biggest challenge facing pittas is to let go of control and apply their powerful will to creating a soft and gentle approach to practice.

Pitta Yoga Series

The pitta yoga series includes plenty of sitting and standing forward bends, which have a cooling and surrendering effect on the body. Most sitting postures are good for pitta individuals, especially bound poses such as Lotus or Reclining Hero, which tend to reduce circulation and refocus the body's attention to the abdomen. This allows for efficient and proper digestion, pitta's major function in the body. Spinal twists and cooling standing postures, such as Triangle, help to drain excess heat from the body.

YOGA FOR PITTAS

PITTA DOSHA

Approach to practice	Cooling, soft, relaxing, forgiving, gentle, diffusive
Vayus to awaken	Samana, apana, prana
Recommended postures	The best postures for pittas promote a playful and noncompetitive attitude. Avoid postures that cause an accumulation of heat.
	Forward bends: Good for pittas, as they are cooling and draw energy to the mid-body
	Spinal twists: Along with forward bends; spinal twists are best for a pitta practice; help to clear the liver and small intestines, areas where pitta accumulates
	Sitting postures: Sitting postures are good, particularly cooling bound postures that stabilize the mid-abdomen region
	Standing postures: Standing postures are beneficial as they promote a downward movement of apana, hence diffusing the heat of the body
	Gentle backbends: Backbends tend to be heating and should be done in moderation; small backbends that release tension from the mid-abdomen are good, such as Cobra, Boat, or Fish pose; accompany backbends with cooling breaths through the mouth
	Inverted postures: Inverted postures tend to be heating in nature and should be avoided or held for short periods
Holds	Moderate to short holds
Areas of concentration	Pitta's site of accumulation: Small intestines
	Other key pitta areas: Mid-abdomen, upper hips, liver, spleen, eyes
Disease tendency	Feverish diseases, infections, inflammatory diseases, diarrhea

The heat is released via the downward flow of apana vayu. Although some backward stretching should be included as a counterforce, deep backbends such as Wheel are heat producing and so should be avoided. This is also true of inversions, such as Headstand, which increase the flow of blood upward, causing an accumulation of heat in the upper extremities and head. Shoulderstand can be practiced in moderation, however, as the bandha at the throat prevents the heating solar energy of the navel from flowing to the head. The cooling pranayama techniques of sithali and sitkari, described in chapter 7, can be combined with heating postures to provide balance.

All postures should be held for a short to moderate length of time, to avoid exertion and heat accumulation. This may disappoint some of you pittas, who love to push yourself to the limit and will settle for nothing less than near perfection. After trying this pitta-calming approach for a while, notice whether that lingering feeling of frustration once experienced following an intense yoga session remains. If you are a pitta individual and leave a yoga class red in the face or with pink splotches on your skin, this is a sign that you are probably overheating yourself. Remember that yoga is a chance to remove ourselves from the competitive world that surrounds us—so relax, let go, and have fun! As we discussed in chapter 3, pitta's main site of accumulation in the body is the small intestines and mid-abdomen. A pitta approach to yoga should therefore draw attention to the abdominal region and aim to balance the body's digestive fire, or agni, which is ruled by pitta. This digestive fire governs the body's ability to metabolize and absorb all of the physical and mental substances consumed by an individual. Other pitta regions of the body that may harbor tensions or sensitivities include the upper hips, liver, spleen, and eyes.

A pitta yoga session should be followed by a final relaxation that is moderate in length, about ten minutes for a ninety-minute yoga session. An eye pillow made of flax seed and lavender helps to cool the pitta mind; cushions placed under the knees can relieve tension in the pelvic region, where pitta tends to accumulate.

Vayus for the Pitta Constitution

As has been previously noted, the most cooling of all the vayus is the linear movement around the abdomen known as samana vayu. When the body's energy is centered around the navel area, it creates a contracting force that channels excess heat into the digestive track for metabolism and absorption.

A pitta yoga practice therefore benefits most from stabilizing postures that increase samana vayu, such as sitting postures and bound poses. One has only to picture the classical Indian posture for eating—sitting cross-legged on the floor in front of a wide banana-leaf plate—to understand how important samana vayu is to the digestive process. Another posture known in India for stimulating digestion is Reclining Hero pose, which is often practiced after completing a meal to help sustain the digestive fire.

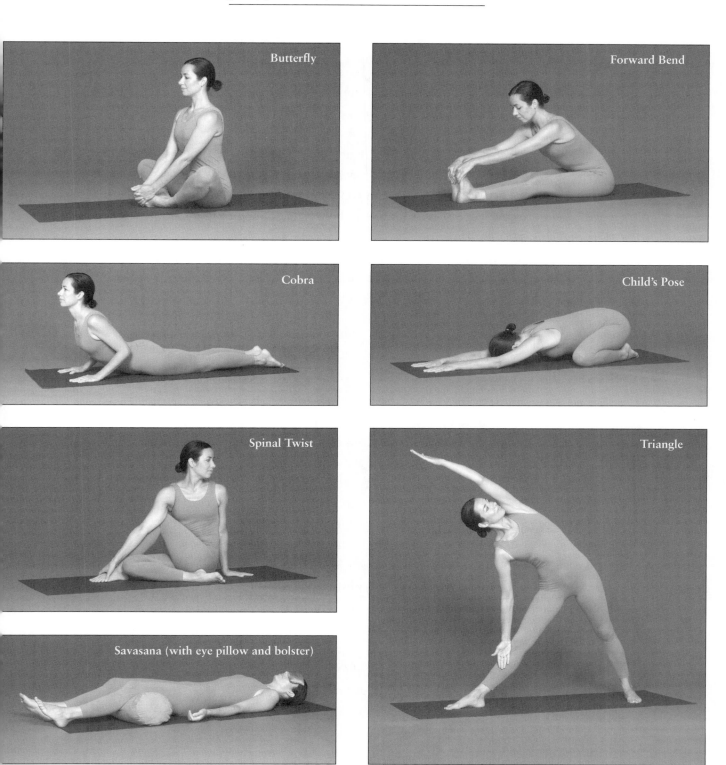

Yoga postures for pittas emphasize forward bends, moderate stretches, and
a cooling and non-competitive approach.

YOGA APPROACH FOR KAPHAS

While vata and pitta individuals need to slow down and relax the body, the already well-relaxed kapha individual benefits from a stimulating yoga approach that is fiery, invigorating, and energizing. Of all the body types, kaphas benefit most from aerobic, heating styles of yoga, such as Bikram, Ashtanga, or Power Yoga. These approaches tend to break up stagnation and release toxins from the body, generating a cleansing process that is highly tonifying for kapha congestion and sluggishness. Postures in this series tend to heat the body, open the chest, develop flexibility, promote blood circulation, and increase heart capacity.

But before entering into a rigorous workout, kaphas should warm up the body properly and proceed with determined effort. Postures should be held for a long period of time, causing some exertion and sweating. The main challenge for kaphas is to muster the willpower to maintain a regular practice—but once they are going they gain much benefit and enjoyment from a regular practice.

Kapha Yoga Series

Kaphas benefit most from postures that promote circulation and mobility and demand more effort from the practitioner. Standing postures wake up the body and counter the kapha tendency toward immobility, inertia, and drowsiness. Backbends are an excellent method of opening the congested kapha chest and increasing circulation from the heart outward to all the extremities. Backbends that are performed on the belly, such as Bow, Boat, or Cobra, are particularly good as they help to stimulate the sluggish kapha digestive fire, which can lead to low metabolism and loss of appetite. Inversions increase the flow of energy to the chest and head, waking up the senses and brain. Spinal twists can help to promote digestion, although standing spinal twists are preferred. Sedentary sitting, prone, or lying postures should be avoided, as they increase the inactivity and stability already well established in kapha types. Forward bends, which contract the chest, may aggravate kapha congestion and should therefore also be avoided.

Kapha's main site of accumulation in the body is the stomach. Other areas of the body that kaphas may want to focus on during a yoga session include the chest, lungs, throat, nose, and sinuses, where mucus tends to accumulate. Yoga postures should aim to open and clear these areas, promoting a discharge of excess mucus.

In contrast to vatas and pittas, kaphas require the shortest period of relaxation after a yoga session. Five to seven minutes of relaxation is sufficient relaxation following a ninety-minute yoga practice. Kaphas will want to use as few pillows and blankets as necessary to avoid falling fast asleep!

YOGA FOR KAPHAS

KAPHA DOSHA

Approach to practice	Stimulating, fiery, aerobic, invigorating, energizing, strenuous, releasing
Vayus to awaken	Udana, vyana
Recommended postures	The best postures for kaphas promote exertion and sweating. Avoid forward bends and sitting postures.
	Standing postures: Excellent for kaphas, especially the more strenuous ones that promote circulation, particularly when combined with long holds and repetition
	Backbends: Promote heating up of the body, open the chest, and increase circulation to the head
	Inversions: Excellent for kaphas, as they increase circulation and an upward flow of energy; they also help to regulate kapha in the area of the chest
	Spinal twists: Standing spinal twists are best for kaphas
	Sitting postures: Increase inertia and therefore should be held for short periods
	Forward bends: Forward bends contract the chest, making this movement less beneficial for kaphas, who can become easily congested.
Holds	Long holds with exertion
Areas of concentration	Kapha's main site of accumulation: Stomach
	Other key kapha areas: Chest, lungs, sinuses, nose, throat, head, joints, pancreas, lymph nodes, synovial fluid
Disease tendency	Respiratory-system diseases, congestion, edema

Vayus for the Kapha Constitution

The stable, earthy nature of kaphas leads to a heavy and stagnant energy flow. For this reason, the vayus that most benefit a kapha practice are those that draw the energy up and out.

The upward movement of udana vayu is activated by inverted postures and poses, in which the arms or legs are raised above the head. This encourages a flow of oxygen and nutrients to the diaphragm, sinuses, and brain. Vyana vayu increases circulation to all parts of the body and is activated by backbends, extensions, and aerobic activities.

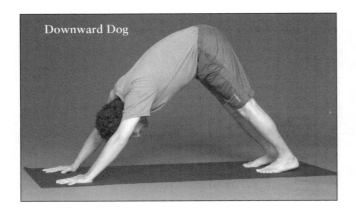
Downward Dog

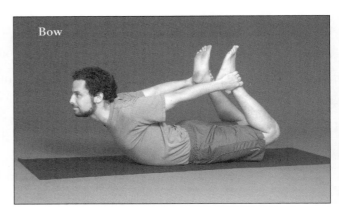
Bow

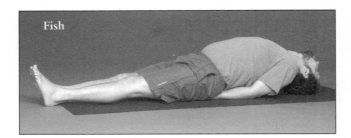
Fish

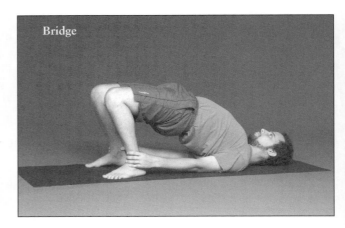
Bridge

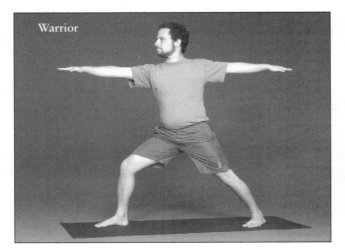
Warrior

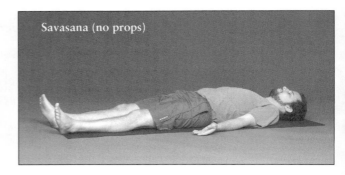
Savasana (no props)

Yoga postures for kaphas emphasize chest-openers, deep backbends, and invigorating standing postures with shorter periods of relaxation.

MEDITATION FOR EACH DOSHA

Within the disciplines of yoga and Ayurveda, meditation is considered the main tool for healing the mind. A regular meditation practice can remove the mental root of the disease process; meditation has the greatest chance of success when the mode is suited to one's doshic type. However, not everyone is ready for meditation; in many cases it may be better to begin with a yoga practice or breathing exercise.

Never try to persuade your recipient to practice a form of meditation that makes him or her uncomfortable, even if you sense that it would be of benefit. If any of your recipients are already well established in a meditation practice, avoid persuading them to change techniques according to their doshic type.

Most importantly, we as practitioners should begin with our own regular meditation practice. A few minutes of metta meditation before seeing a client will clear the mind and facilitate a positive healing energy in the room. The transmission of thoughts of loving-kindness helps to counter any judgments or negative thinking, enabling us to become more effective tools of Ayurveda.

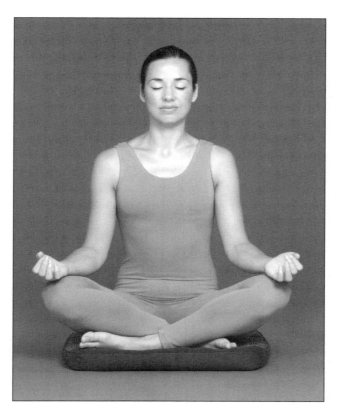

A few minutes of metta meditation before seeing a client helps to clear the mind.

MEDITATION FOR EACH DOSHA

 VATA

Approach	Grounded form of meditation, such as mantra repetition, observation of silence, or visualization
Mantras	Warm, soft, soothing, and calming mantras, such as *Om, Ram,* and *Hum*

 PITTA

Approach	Self-inquiry techniques such as Vedanta, Zen, and Vipassana
Mantras	Cool, soothing, and calming mantras such as *Om, Aim, Shrim,* and *Sham*

 KAPHA

Approach	Bhakti path of chanting, singing, and prayer or the karma yoga path of volunteer and charity work
Mantras	Warm, stimulating, and energizing mantras such as *Om, Hum,* and *Aim*

Calming the Vata Mind

One of the key challenges for vatas is to concentrate the mind, as the abundance of air in the vata constitution can lead to daydreaming and worry. It is important for these individuals to enjoy the present moment and to gently bring the mind back to the breath when it begins to wander. Maintaining a regular meditation practice at the same hour and location every day can be a tremendous help in this effort. Vata persons require a grounded form of meditation, such as mantra repetition, observation of silence, or visualization. This will help them to cultivate positive seeds of faith and remove the doubt, worry, anxiety, and fear that tends to torment vata individuals. *Trataka,* concentration on one object, such as a steady flame, is particularly good for restless vatas in helping the mind to become one-pointed.

The powerful seed mantras of *Om, Ram,* and *Hum* are known to be especially grounding for vatas. Whenever your vata client appears to be out of balance, you may instruct them to vocally chant these mantras for a minute, and then repeat them silently. It is also useful to burn grounding and strengthening fragrances, such as patchouli, musk, myrrh, or cinnamon, or to play soothing music.

Cooling the Pitta Mind

The best form of meditation for pitta types is one that softens the mind and allows for the growth of compassion, forgiveness, and overall release. Although the sharp pitta mind excels at analysis and critical thinking, these types need to work on opening the heart, releasing anger, and letting go of control. Self-inquiry meditation techniques, such as Vedanta, Zen, and Vipassana, are recommended. Pitta individuals often have good concentration and can meditate easily, but they must take care not to turn meditation into an ambition venture.

These types should focus on cultivating peace, love, forgiveness, being noncompetitive, and leaving all judgments and frustrations aside. The yoga seed mantras that create a cool, soothing effect on the spirit are *Om, Aim, Shrim,* and *Sham.* The most suitable fragrance for balancing pitta is the sweet, cooling smell of sandalwood, which is applied to the forehead as a purification gesture before entering a temple in the blazing heat of India. Other sweet fragrances are found in the scent of flowers, including jasmine, rose, gardenia, lotus, and lavender.

Awakening the Kapha Mind

One of the greatest challenges facing kapha individuals is getting started with a regular meditation or yoga practice. The best mental approach for individuals of this nature is one that focuses on reaching established goals and maintaining a predetermined practice. The kapha tendency toward drowsiness can be countered by an unwavering determination to keep going, which becomes easier as the benefits of the practice begin to emerge. Meditating in groups can also help motivate these individuals.

Kapha individuals benefit from the *bhakti* devotional path of meditation, which includes chanting, singing, reading spiritual texts, and praying. Also recommended is the active meditation of *karma yoga,* or selflessly helping others through volunteer or charity work. While practicing meditation, kaphas should focus on breaking away from material comforts, attachment, and sentimentality. The mantra sounds of *Om, Hum,* and *Aim* can be repeated mentally or vocally to create a warm, stimulating, and energizing effect on the body.

Chanting and singing in general are highly beneficial for kaphas, as they create vibrations in the lungs and sinuses and wake up the mind. Warming and stimulating fragrances, such as camphor, eucalyptus, sage, and mint, may help to maintain focus and alertness.

Yoga and meditation are powerful practices that have traditionally played an important therapeutic role within the ancient science of Ayurveda. When practiced according to the doshic needs of each individual, these techniques have the potential to restore balance, increase mental clarity, and facilitate spiritual growth. It is not necessary to make an appointment or spend a lot of money to practice yoga or meditation—all that is required is a quiet room and a mat.

By sharing basic yoga and meditation recommendations with our recipients, the healing potential of our Thai Yoga Therapy practice expands beyond the massage room.

Now let's consider how to enhance wellness through another ancient pillar of Ayurvedic medicine—nutrition and diet.

16

Food and Vitality: Ayurvedic Nutrition

In India there is an old adage that states "the cupboard is your medicine cabinet." This simple statement captures a uniquely Ayurvedic perspective on food and nutrition: that everything we eat has the potential to heal or harm us. In Ayurveda, nutrition accounts for about fifty percent of all treatments, demonstrating the incredible power of food when directed in the correct way. This is hard to communicate within our Western culture, where eating is often regarded as an indulgence and driven by unhealthy cravings. With excessive quantities of salt, sugar, artificial flavors, additives, and preservatives, much of the food in the Western diet overstimulates and drains the body. Unfortunately, with the fast speed of modern life many people find themselves with little time or energy to prepare and enjoy healthy, balanced meals together with friends and family. This is an indicator of the imbalance of our society as a whole, and reveals a tendency that we should aim to move away from in our daily lives. Eating an Ayurvedic diet *does* take more time than ordering a pizza or preparing frozen foods, but it can be a great force for achieving greater equilibrium in our lives. There is nothing more nurturing than preparing a wholesome, delicious meal for yourself or your loved ones.

In this chapter we will introduce you to some straightforward principles of Ayurvedic nutrition that you can gradually integrate into your life and share with your clients.

The first step to finding a balanced diet begins with understanding your unique doshic constitution. Each doshic type requires a different approach to nutrition, the food choices acting as a counterbalance to the predominant qualities in your individual nature. For example, a light-framed, cool vata would benefit from a warming diet that is grounding, substantial, and highly nutritious. The heavy, immobile kapha, on the other hand, best benefits from a light, spicy diet that stimulates digestion and mobilizes all of the bodily systems.

By gaining an understanding of these subtle differences, the act of eating becomes a sacred vehicle for achieving optimum health. We are what we eat, but we are also *how* we eat. The location, quantity, pace, and mental state in which we consume food is just as important as the amount of protein or vitamins we receive per serving. According to Ayurveda, when healthy, wholesome food is taken properly there is no need for supplemental vitamins. All the nutrients we require are already in the food and it is better to receive them in a pure and natural form.

Before considering the basic nutritional approach recommended for each dosha, let's look at some general principles for healthy eating according to Ayurveda.

TEN PRINCIPLES OF HEALTHY EATING

Over 2500 years ago the Ayurvedic sage Charaka laid down ten fundamental principles for healthy eating. At that time there were no over-the-counter digestive aids to counteract the negative effects of an imbalanced meal. As a result, proper nutrition was revered as the main source of disease prevention and longevity.

We have outlined Charaka's ten precepts here, modifying and elaborating upon them to suit modern times.

1. Do not eat too much or too little.

Consuming the appropriate quantity of food is an essential component to Ayurvedic nutrition. To measure the correct quantity of food, place your hands together with your palms facing upward to form a bowl. This cup, called an *anjali,* tells us how much each of us can individually consume. According to Ayurveda, one should refrain from exceeding more than two *anjalis* in one sitting.

During a meal, avoid filling the stomach to its full capacity, as this disables the function of the gastric muscles and suffocates the digestive fire of agni. Ayurveda recommends filling the stomach 50 percent with solids and 25 percent with liquids, and then leaving the final 25 percent empty. The liquid foods combine with the gastric enzymes in the stomach to form a digestive potion that essentially "cooks" the solid foods, allowing for efficient digestion.

Allowing for some empty space provides room for the food to be churned in preparation for digestion. Students often ask us how you know that you have one-quarter of empty space in your stomach. The exact ratio is not important; what matters most is that you stop consuming before you feel overly full. This requires tuning into our bodies and eating for nutrition, rather than indulging every craving that arises.

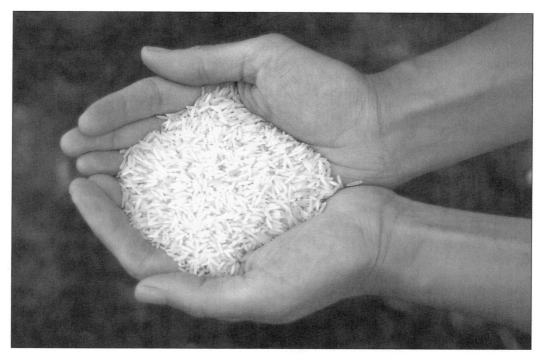

Anjali mudra is a measurement created by joining two hands to form an empty bowl.
Ayurveda tells us to refrain from consuming more than two anjalis in one sitting.

2. Warm, well-cooked foods are best.

According to Ayurveda, cooked or semi-cooked foods are already partially digested and therefore require less energy to fully digest. For this reason, warm, prepared foods such as stews, soups, or sauces are generally preferred to raw foods. This nutritional principle is shared throughout much of the Asian world, where eating a salad or cold sandwich is often met with curiosity and disbelief. Simmering foods in spices and combining compatible food types generally increases overall digestibility and nutritional value.

3. Fresh, tasty, whole grains and organic foods are best.

One of the greatest challenges of eating Ayurvedically today is the omnipresent supply of canned, frozen, freeze-dried, genetically modified, processed, preserved, and hormone- and pesticide-laden foods. All of these procedures drain food products of their natural levels of prana, the subtle life force that provides us with energy, vitality, and general well-being. Stale, leftover foods also contain lower levels of prana. As much as possible, use fresh, organic produce in cooking and regularly restock your cupboards with whole grains, spices, and legumes. Choose whole grains over refined products, such as white flours and sugars.

4. Never rush eating.

Ayurveda believes that every morsel of food that we consume is a sacred offering from Mother Nature. For this reason, eating is considered a sanctified ritual that requires our full awareness. If we do not pay attention while eating, our bodies will not pay attention while digesting. Every bite should be chewed thoroughly to activate the digestive enzymes in our saliva in preparation for digestion. Create a peaceful environment for eating in your home, a place where you will be undisturbed by television, radio, or excessive chatter. When possible, try eating in silence and begin your meal with a prayer.

5. Eat in more than eating out.

Many of us have access to an assortment of restaurants with delicious fare from all over the world. While this is certainly appealing in many ways, Ayurveda recommends eating the majority of our meals at home. Restaurants cater to a mass audience and are usually forced to rely on canned, frozen, and preserved ingredients that contain high quantities of salt and fat. Perhaps most importantly, restaurant foods are made for commercial reasons and therefore lack the intention of home-cooked meals prepared in a loving and nurturing environment.

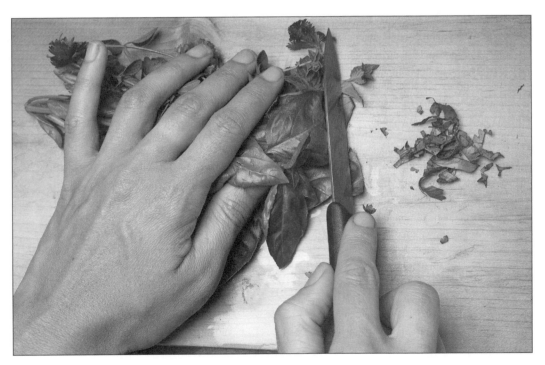

When practiced with full awareness in the present moment,
cooking becomes a form of meditation.

6. Avoid snacking.

Food is best eaten on an empty stomach, after your last meal has been digested. Ayurveda advises a period of four to six hours between meals and as little snacking as possible. Fruits are an ideal snack for all three doshas, and vatas can indulge in light snacking to sustain their variable energy. Wait at least two hours after a meal before either sleeping or exercising.

7. Eat compatible foods.

As a general rule, foods should work together; they should not contradict one another in their actions. Avoid combining foods with widely divergent properties—for example, do not combine cold foods with hot foods or light foods with heavy foods. The combination of raw foods and cooked foods is avoided in Ayurveda.

8. Switch to a vegetarian diet.

According to Ayurveda, animal flesh is considered difficult to digest; it is heavy, and so is tamasic in nature. Animals are imbued with their own consciousness and karmic energy. We ingest that energy when we eat meat. When we eat meat, we are consuming the fear that is felt by animals pent up in cages and waiting for slaughter. We are also consuming the high levels of hormones and antibiotics pumped into their systems. Ayurveda follows the Vedic tradition of *ahimsa,* the avoidance of harming any living creature. Except for rare cases of debilitation, Ayurveda prescribes a vegetarian diet for all healthy individuals.

9. Drink an adequate amount of water.

Water should be sipped in small quantities during your meal, but never directly before or after your meal, as this will lower the digestive fire of *agni.* Another tip for keeping your agni burning high is to avoid ice, which puts out the digestive fire. As Dr. Vasant Lad says in his Ayurvedic training courses, "ice is not nice!" Water should be consumed regularly throughout the day, not gulped down in large quantities. Vatas require the most amount of daily water intake (seven to ten glasses), pittas are in the middle (five to six glasses), and kaphas require the least amount (four to five glasses).

10. Avoid eating after sunset.

A final principle of Ayurvedic nutrition is to avoid eating after sunset. This can be quite difficult to accomplish in the winter season, especially in the north, where it gets dark by 4 PM, but we should generally avoid eating heavy meals late at night. Consuming large meals before going to sleep creates a sluggish digestive system and increases mucous in the body.

EATING FOR YOUR DOSHA

The key principles outlined above provide a good start to healthy eating, but to achieve optimal balance it is recommended that you follow a diet designed for your doshic type. According to Ayurveda, you should eat foods that are nourishing for your particular constitution and that suit your mental and emotional temperament. Every food item that we put into our mouths is endowed with certain qualities, which can be used to either balance or disrupt our doshic makeup. Following the simple but sage rule of thumb that opposites heal each other, Ayurveda uses nutrition to counterbalance doshic imbalances. For example, if you are a red-headed, feisty pitta, you should avoid foods that increase your fiery temperament—foods such as chili peppers, garlic, raw onions, and deep-fried foods. Cooling, calming foods, such as sweet fruits, fresh greens, basmati rice, and dairy products, would be more suitable. This easy, straightforward approach to nutrition forces us to become aware of the qualities and content of the foods that we are consuming. You will be surprised at how customizing your diet according to your doshic type can provide comfort and lead to a stronger and overall better digestive system.

In order to gain an understanding of how to eat for your constitution, let's look at the general nutritional approach for each dosha. If you are a dual or triple type, you would follow dietary recommendations in order to calm the dosha that you feel is causing the most imbalance in your body.

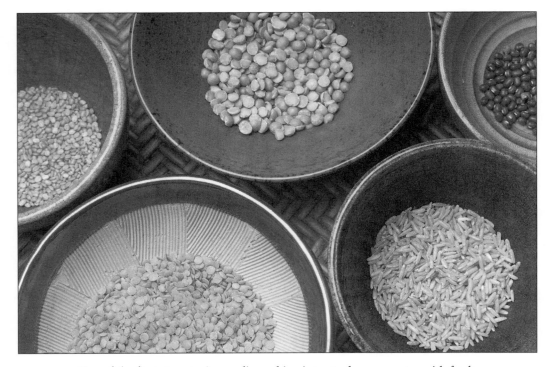

One of the first steps to Ayurvedic cooking is to stock your pantry with fresh,
organic whole grains and legumes.

Vata Diet

Persons of a vata nature should follow a diet that is moist, calming, warming, and highly nourishing. These qualities counterbalance the cool, dry, airlike mobility that causes vata individuals to feel ungrounded, nervous, and cold. Well-cooked whole grains with root vegetable stews and lightly spiced curries and sauces help to ground and stabilize vata. Basmati rice, brown rice, wild rice, oatmeal, and wheat pastas are excellent, as are well-cooked split mung beans and soy beans. Moderate amounts of spices that warm the body and aid digestion should be used, including cumin, cinnamon, cardamom, ginger, nutmeg, and black pepper.

For vatas, food should be moistening, with plenty of oil or ghee to aid digestion and lubricate the skin and the internal organs. Most dairy and soy products are grounding for vata, as are sweet and sour fruits. Of all the doshas, vatas require the most healthy fats to build up the body, which can be acquired in the form of oils, nuts, avocados, and dairy products, and in organic meats for nonvegetarians. Cold, raw, and greasy foods aggravate the sensitive vata digestion, as does any form of fast food or junk food.

Meals should be small and frequent, but regular and taken in a calming environment without external stimulation. Meals should not be eaten when a vata person is excessively worried, nervous, or afraid, as this will only cause further imbalance. The recommended tastes for vata include sweet, sour, and mildly salty, with a moderate use of pungent spices.

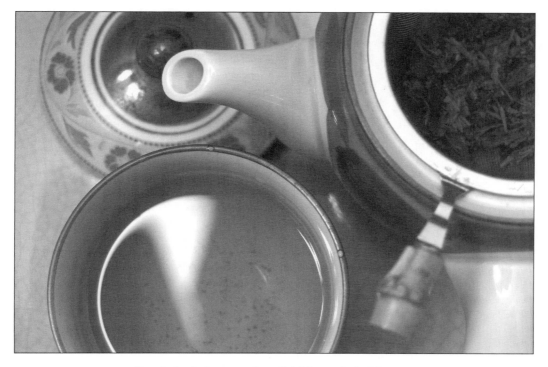

Certain herbal teas are beneficial for each doshic type.

Pitta Diet

Pittas require a diet that is cool, slightly dry, and a little heavy. In the summer, a wide variety of raw foods should be taken, while warmer cooked foods spiced with cumin, coriander, or fennel are better in the winter. Cool grains such as basmati rice, wheat, barley, breads, rice cakes, and crackers are highly beneficial. Goat, cow, and soy milk are effective in cooling pitta, as are cottage cheese, soft cheeses, and tofu. Most vegetables, fresh greens, and salads are recommended, as are sweet and astringent fruits.

Of all the doshas, pitta requires the most protein, attainable in the form of tofu, mung beans, dairy products, and whole wheat grains, and from organic poultry and moderate amounts of fish for nonvegetarians. Although it is sometimes difficult for the passionate pitta type, it is essential to avoid fried foods, spicy foods, and overstimulation through alcohol, red meat, caffeine, and cigarettes.

In order to cater to the strong pitta appetite and avoid irritability, meals should be taken regularly three times a day; meals should never be skipped. Steer clear of late-night snacking or eating when feeling angry, frustrated, or upset. The recommended tastes for pittas include sweet, bitter, and astringent.

Kapha Diet

Individuals of a kapha nature benefit most from foods that are warm, light, and dry in nature. Recommended grains include quinoa, soba noodles, millet, rye, and oat bran. Light low-fat proteins, high-fiber beans, and generous portions of vegetables with pungent spices are excellent. Astringent and bitter fruits are good, as are light and crispy foods such as steamed vegetables, salads, popcorn, and corn tortillas.

Kapha types may love sweet, creamy foods, but these are the most aggravating for their constitution. They should avoid cold, heavy, and oily products such as ice cream, creamy yogurt, deep-fried foods, and meat. Pungent spices such as ginger, garlic, black pepper, and cayenne help to break up mucous and increase agni, the digestive fire that is naturally low in kapha types (resulting in sluggish digestion).

Three small meals a day, with the biggest meal at noon is the best nutritional schedule for stimulating kapha digestion. Allow at least three to four hours between meals and avoid eating after 6 PM. Kaphas should also be aware of a tendency to use eating as an emotional support or comfort during times of difficulty. The recommended tastes for kapha types include pungent, astringent, and bitter.

The Ayurvedic Food Guidelines chart on pages 173 to 176 provides a detailed list of food recommendations for each body type. This is not meant to be a rigid guideline but rather a general overview of the foods one may wish to increase or avoid, based on the predominant quality of that food.

AYURVEDIC FOOD GUIDELINES

VATA

PITTA

KAPHA

FRUITS

Yes: *sweet and sour*	No: *astringent or dried*	Yes: *sweet*	No: *sour*	Yes: *astringent or dried*	No: *sweet*
apples (cooked)	apples (raw)	apples (sweet)	apples (sour)	apples	avocado
apricots	cranberries	apricots	bananas	apricots	bananas
avocado	pears	berries	cranberries	berries	coconut
bananas	pomegranate	cherries	grapefruit	cranberries	dates
berries	prunes (dry)	coconut	grapes (green)	figs	figs
cherries	raisins (dry)	dates	lemon	grapes*	grapefruit*
coconut		figs	mangos*	lemon*, lime*	kiwi
grapefruit		grapes (red)	oranges (sour)	mangos*	melons
grapes		lime*	papaya*	peaches*	oranges
kiwi		melons	rhubarb	pears*	papaya
lemon, lime		oranges (sweet)		pomegranate	pineapple
mangos		peaches		prunes	plums
melons		pears		raisins	watermelon
oranges		pineapple		strawberries*	
papaya		plums (sweet)			
peaches		pomegranate			
pineapple		prunes			
plums		strawberries*			
rhubarb		watermelon			

VEGETABLES

Yes: *sweet, cooked, root vegetables*	No: *astringent, raw*	Yes: *astringent, bitter*	No: *sour, pungent*	Yes: *astringent, pungent*	No: *sweet, moist*
asparagus	artichoke	artichoke	beets	artichoke	cucumber
beets	bell pepper*	asparagus	carrots (raw)*	asparagus	eggplant*
carrots	broccoli*	bell pepper*	chili pepper	beets	okra
cucumber*	cabbage*	broccoli	corn*	bell pepper	parsnip*
green beans	cauliflower*	cabbage	eggplant*	broccoli	potatoes*
leafy greens	celery	cauliflower	garlic	cabbage	spinach*
(cooked)	eggplant*	celery	mustard greens	carrots	squash*
okra	kale	cucumber	onions	cauliflower	sweet potatoes*
onions (cooked)	leafy greens	green beans	parsley*	celery	tomatoes
parsley	(raw)	kale	radish	corn	(raw)*
parsnip	mushrooms	leafy greens	spinach*	green beans	water chestnuts
radish	peas*	lettuce	tomatoes*	kale	zucchini*
spinach*	potatoes*	mushrooms	turnip*	leafy greens	
squash	sprouts*	okra		mushrooms	
(summer)	tomatoes	radicchio		onions	
sweet potatoes	(raw)*	peas		parsley	
turnip		potatoes		peas	
zucchini*		sprouts		radish	
		sweet potatoes		sprouts	
		watercress*		turnip	
		zucchini			

*These foods are okay in moderation.

	VATA		PITTA		KAPHA
GRAINS: *WHOLE GRAINS RECOMMENDED FOR ALL TYPES*					
Yes	No: *avoid dry grains and yeasted breads*	Yes	No: *avoid yeasted breads in excess*	Yes: *dry, whole grains*	No: *avoid bread*

amaranth*
 basmati rice
 brown rice
 bulgur*
 oats
 quinoa
 wheat
   couscous*
 whole wheat
	barley*
	 buckwheat*
	 cereals (dry)
	 corn*
	 corn chips
	 couscous
	 granola
	 millet*
	 rye*
	 spelt
	 white flour
		amaranth
		 barley
		 basmati rice
		 bulgur
		 couscous
		 granola
		 oats
		 spelt
		 unyeasted
		   breads
		 whole wheat
			brown rice*
			 buckwheat
			 corn*
			 millet*
			 rye*
			 white flour
				amaranth*
				 barley
				 basmati rice
				 buckwheat
				 cereal
				 corn
				 couscous
				 millet*
				 oat bran
				 quinoa*
				 rye
				 spelt*
				 wheat bran
					oats
					 pasta*
					 rice*
					 rice cakes*
					 sweet granola*
					 wheat
					 white flour

LEGUMES					
Yes	No	Yes: *most beans are ok*	No	Yes: *all beans are generally good*	No
aduki beans* lentils (red) lima beans* mung beans mung dal peanuts* soy tofu*	black beans chick peas fava beans kidney beans navy beans pinto beans split peas	aduki beans chick peas lentils (all) mung beans mung dal tempeh tofu	miso toor dal	black beans chick peas lentils (all) mung beans mung dal soy milk split peas tempeh tofu (hot)*	kidney beans soy tofu (cold)
NUTS/SEEDS					
Yes: *all nuts/ seeds good in moderation*	No	Yes	No: *avoid most nuts, as they are too heating for pitta*	Yes	No: *avoid most nuts/seeds*

almonds
   (soaked)
 pumpkin seeds
 sesame seeds
 sunflower seeds
	popcorn
	 psyllium seeds*
		almonds
		   (soaked)*
		 coconut
		 flax seeds
		 psyllium seeds
		 pumpkin seeds*
		 sunflower seeds
				popcorn
				 poppy seeds
				 pumpkin seeds*
				 sunflower seeds	

OILS					
Yes: *all oils are generally good*	No:	Yes: *avoid in excess*	No:	Yes: *take in small quantities*	No: *use oil sparingly*
almond ghee olive sesame	flax seed*	canola coconut ghee flax seed* olive* soy sunflower	almond* apricot corn mustard safflower sesame	canola corn ghee* safflower soy sunflower	

VATA		PITTA		KAPHA	
DAIRY PRODUCTS					
Yes: *most dairy is good, particularly sour products*	No	Yes	No	Yes	No
butter buttermilk cottage cheese kefir milk soft cheese yogurt (spiced)	hard cheese* powdered milk	butter (unsalted) cottage cheese cream cheese ice cream milk soft cheese yogurt (diluted)*	buttermilk* feta kefir* salty and hard cheese sour cream	buttermilk* cottage cheese goat's milk soy milk yogurt (low-fat or diluted)*	butter cheese of all kinds ice cream milk sour cream
SWEET					
Yes: *all-natural sweeteners good in moderation*	No	Yes: *all-natural sweeteners good in moderation*	No	Yes	No: *avoid most sweeteners, especially white sugar*
honey molasses	white sugar		honey* molasses white sugar	raw honey	
HERBS/SPICES					
Yes	No	Yes: *avoid hot spices*	No	Yes: *the spicier the better!*	No
all spice anise asafoetida basil bay leaves black pepper* cardamom cilantro cinnamon cloves coriander cumin fennel garlic ginger (fresh) licorice marjoram mint* mustard seeds nutmeg orange peel oregano paprika saffron sage tarragon thyme turmeric	cayenne* dill* fenugreek* salt*	basil (fresh) black pepper* caraway* cardamom* cilantro cinnamon coriander cumin dill fennel ginger (fresh) gotu kola lemon grass licorice mint orange peel* saffron turmeric vanilla*	allspice asafoetida basil (dry)* bay leaves cayenne cloves garlic ginger (dry) fenugreek marjoram mustard seeds nutmeg oregano paprika rosemary sage salt* thyme	all spice anise asafoetida bay leaves basil black pepper cardamom cayenne chilies cilantro cinnamon coriander cumin fennel* fenugreek garlic ginger (fresh) lemon grass marjoram mint mustard seeds nutmeg orange peel oregano paprika saffron sage tarragon turmeric	licorice salt* vanilla*

VATA		PITTA		KAPHA	
BEVERAGES: *ALL THREE TYPES SHOULD AVOID ICED DRINKS*					
Yes	No	Yes	No	Yes	No
almond milk	alcohol (hard)	almond milk	alcohol (hard)	apple juice*	alcohol (hard)
apple cider	apple juice	apple juice	caffeine	berry juice	almond milk
beer*	caffeine	beer*	carbonated	carrot juice	beer
chai	carbonated	chai*	drinks	chai	dairy drinks
grape juice	drinks	dairy drinks	red wine	cranberry juice	lemonade
orange juice	cold dairy	rice milk	sour juices	prune juice	rice milk
rice milk	cranberry juice	soy milk		soy milk	orange juice
soy milk		sweet juices		(warm)	sweet juices
(warm)				wine (dry)*	wine (sweet)
white wine*					
HERB TEAS					
Yes	No	Yes	No	Yes	No
anise	dandelion	alfalfa	cinnamon	blackberry	licorice*
cardamom	ginseng	blackberry	clove	cardamom	marshmallow
chamomile	hibiscus	chamomile	ginger (dry)	chamomile	rosehips*
cinnamon	jasmine*	coriander	ginseng	cinnamon	
fennel	nettle*	cumin		eucalyptus	
ginger (fresh)	red clover*	fennel		fennel	
ginseng		ginger (fresh)		hyssop	
licorice		hibiscus		orange peel	
orange peel		jasmine		peppermint	
peppermint		raspberry			

THE SIX TASTES OF AYURVEDA

The recommended guidelines of nutrition in Ayurveda are scientifically designed according to the system of the six tastes, or the *rasas*, of sweet, salty, sour, astringent, pungent, and bitter. *Rasa* is a Sanskrit word with many meanings. In addition to taste, *rasa* refers to plasma, the first of the seven bodily tissues that feeds all the other tissues. *Rasa* also means "emotion," reflecting the Ayurvedic belief that our mental state is directly connected to the food that we consume. We are what we eat—on a physical, mental, and spiritual level.

Let us now review each of the six tastes in more detail to gain a clearer understanding of the reasoning behind the dietary choices recommended by Ayurveda.

Sweet rasa (earth and water)   Recommended for: Vata and pitta

The majority of the food that we consume has a sweet rasa; some researchers put the figure as high as 70 to 75 percent. This does not refer to the sugary sweet taste

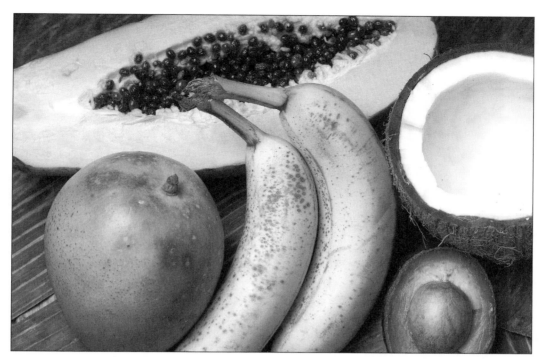

Most fruits and vegetables carry the sweet rasa, as do the majority of foods we consume.

we often think of in the West. The sweet rasa is the natural, wholesome sweetness of fruits, vegetables, and unprocessed grains. The sweet rasa operates as a staple taste of nourishment, creation, and growth. It enhances the bodily forces of immunity, strength, and vitality, or *ojas*. Sweetness is critical during childhood, while the body is undergoing rapid growth and development. The sweet taste, in moderation, encourages proper functioning of the senses, improves the complexion, relieves burning sensations, promotes healthy tissue growth, and enhances an overall sweetness of the mind.

The sweet rasa is composed of earth and water, which makes it similar to the kapha dosha in many ways. Like kapha, the sweet taste is very heavy and wet. It is neutral in temperature and can be cooling or heating, depending on the specific food product. For example, honey and maple syrup are both sweet in taste, but maple syrup is more cooling while honey is heating. Due to its similarity with kapha, the sweet taste tends to increase kapha and reduce vata and pitta.

Examples of foods carrying the sweet rasa include most dairy products, particularly milk, soft cheeses, ghee, butter, and ice cream. Most fruits and vegetables are sweet, as are the majority of grains, including rice, wheat, bran, and oats. Legumes and beans are sweet, as are most animal products, including red meat, poultry, and eggs.

THE SIX TASTES OF AYURVEDA

RASA (TASTE)	ELEMENT	BALANCES	AGGRAVATES (IN EXCESS)
sweet	earth + water	vata, pitta	kapha
salty	water + fire	vata	kapha, pitta
sour (acid)	earth + fire	vata	pitta, kapha
astringent	air + earth	kapha, pitta	vata
pungent	fire + air	kapha	pitta, vata
bitter	air + ether	pitta, kapha	vata

Salty rasa (water and fire)   Recommended for: Vata

The salty rasa, made up of water and fire, shares many qualities with pitta. Like pitta, the salty taste is heating and moist in nature. The salty rasa softens the bodily tissues and promotes waste elimination, but in excess it can lead to water retention and bloating. Salt is anti-flatulent, provides muscle strength, and stimulates salivation, which aids in digestion and absorption. The salty taste has a soothing effect on vata, but it can increase pitta and kapha.

This taste is related to the natural saltiness that occurs in sea salt, mineral salt, rock salt, soy sauce, seafood, and seaweed. According to Ayurveda, mineral rock salt is highly recommended, as it contains many minerals in addition to sodium.

Sour rasa (earth and fire)   Recommended for: Vata

The sour rasa is composed of earth and fire, making it a stabilizing and heating taste. Sour tastes tend to be oily and liquid in nature; they stimulate metabolism. The acidic quality of sour stimulates the secretion of digestive enzymes and eliminates congestion. However, in excess sour dries the membranes and can lead to hyperacidity, heartburn, acid indigestion, or diarrhea in pitta types. While sour can increase pitta and kapha, it is very balancing for vata, but it should be taken in small doses due to its powerful effect.

The sour rasa is found in sour fruits such as grapefruit, oranges, mangos, lemons, limes, and green grapes. Tomatoes, vinegar, yogurt, sour cream, cheese, and fermented foods such as miso are further examples of the sour rasa. This taste is known for improving appetite and aiding with digestion and waste elimination.

Astringent rasa (air and earth) Recommended for: Kapha and pitta

The astringent rasa is composed of the air and earth elements; it is cooling, drying, and heavy in nature. This taste is anti-inflammatory, decongestive, and fat reducing. It is useful for binding the stool in cases of diarrhea and blood clotting. In excess, the astringent rasa can cause dryness in various parts of the body that manifest as constipation, infertility, emaciation, and dryness in the mouth or throat. The astringent rasa is beneficial for drying out kapha and cooling down pitta, but can aggravate vata due to its light and dry qualities.

Examples of foods containing the astringent rasa include raw vegetables, sprouts, bell peppers, broccoli, plantains, green beans, celery, and leafy greens such as lettuce, bok choy, and spinach. Astringent can also be found in fruits such as apples, pomegranates, unripe bananas, and berries. Many dried legumes are astringent, such as chick peas, lentils, and split peas. Herbal, black, and green teas are astringent, as are some spices, including turmeric, nutmeg, poppy seeds, and sage.

Pungent rasa (fire and air)   Recommended for: Kapha

The pungent rasa contains the fire and air elements, and is therefore hot, light, and dry in nature. These are qualities very much needed by kapha types, who are cool, heavy, and wet. In moderation, the pungent rasa kindles the digestive fire of agni and promotes proper absorption. Pungent also increases circulation and clears stagnation in the body as it appears in the form of congestion, blood clots, or excess fat. In abundance, the pungent rasa can lead to diarrhea, heartburn, ulcers, insomnia, inflammation, and irritability.

Pungent is especially beneficial for kaphas and can be taken by vatas in moderation. The heating, light qualities of pungent aggravates pitta types.

The pungent taste is found in much of our favorite cooking ingredients, such as chili peppers, garlic, ginger, and onions. Many spices are pungent in nature such as black pepper, mustard, bay leaf, oregano, and cayenne. Some vegetables with the pungent taste include radish, mustard greens, beets (raw), carrots, parsley, spinach, Swiss chard, turnips, and cabbage.

Bitter rasa (air and ether)   Recommended for: Pitta and kapha

Like the vata dosha, bitter is made up of the air and ether elements, making it cold, dry, and light in nature. The bitter rasa has anti-inflammatory qualities, and it purifies toxins and reduces fat in the body, but excessive consumption of this rasa can cause extreme dryness, emaciation, and fatigue. The bitter rasa has a neutralizing effect on the senses, reducing excessive cravings and urges—bitter is used by spiritual celibates in India to reduce sexual energies.

Following the Ayurvedic rule of thumb that like increases like, the bitter taste increases vata in the body and should therefore be avoided by most vata individuals. Its cool properties pacify pitta and its dryness reduces kapha.

RELATIONSHIPS AMONG THE SIX RASAS

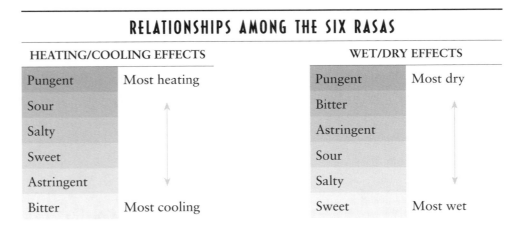

HEATING/COOLING EFFECTS		WET/DRY EFFECTS	
Pungent	Most heating	Pungent	Most dry
Sour		Bitter	
Salty		Astringent	
Sweet		Sour	
Astringent		Salty	
Bitter	Most cooling	Sweet	Most wet

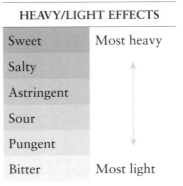

HEAVY/LIGHT EFFECTS	
Sweet	Most heavy
Salty	
Astringent	
Sour	
Pungent	
Bitter	Most light

Bitter is the least common taste available in the Western diet, perhaps due to its neutralizing and unstimulating effects. Some examples of bitter vegetables now available in the West include bitter melon, bitter gourd, rapine, radicchio, bitter cucumber, and dandelion root. Bitter is also found in coffee and aloe vera and in some uncommon herbs, such as yellow dock, sandalwood, neem, turmeric, and fenugreek.

SEVEN STEPS TO AN AYURVEDIC KITCHEN

In order to effectively integrate Ayurveda into our daily diet, we must have the proper working space with all of the necessary tools and ingredients. Below you will find seven practical steps that will help you transform your kitchen into a sacred Ayurvedic space.

1. Update your spice rack.
Spices have a shelf life of about six to twelve months, after which time they begin to lessen in taste and medicinal value. For this reason it is advisable to purchase spices in small quantities. If you have the time you can roast the seeds and grind them yourself.

Here are the spices you will find most useful.

asafoetida	fennel seeds
basil	ginger (dried)
cardamom pods (green)	bay leaves
cardamom powder	mustard seeds (brown)
cayenne	nutmeg
cinnamon	oregano
cloves	black pepper corns
coriander seeds and powder	salt (mineral or sea)
cumin seeds and powder	thyme
curry powder	turmeric

2. Stock your pantry.
Here are some items that you might want to have in your pantry or accessible at a local market.

ginger (fresh)	chick peas (dried)
garlic (fresh)	white sesame seeds
coriander (fresh)	raisins
green chilies (not for pittas!)	tamari
brown rice	sesame oil
basmati rice	raw honey
red lentils	ghee (clarified butter)
mung dal	jaggary sugar

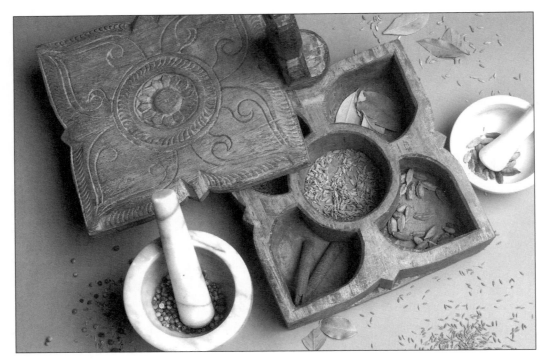

In India, cooking spices are considered highly therapeutic and
traditionally kept in a decorative wooden box.

3. Clean out your supply.

Ayurveda believes that frozen and canned foods are considered to be less nutritional and
lacking in prana. As much as possible, remove all frozen, canned, preserved, and processed
foods from your kitchen. In general, frozen foods are preferred to canned items, but they
are still a distant second to freshly prepared foods. Prepared, frozen, or canned meals are
low in prana and tend to contain high levels of sodium and artificial ingredients.

4. Eat organically.

Due to the increased use of pesticides and hormones in our foods, it is advisable to use
organic products when possible, especially when using soy and dairy products, and
meats. Use naturally processed oils, rather than hydrogenated or commercial brands,
and produce that is seasonal and organic.

5. Eat whole grains.

Replace the grains in your diet with whole grain items such as whole wheat bread,
cereal, or pasta, brown rice, or whole grain oatmeal. Other healthy options include
cracked wheat bulgur or buckwheat, whole wheat couscous, and whole grain corn,
rye, or barley. This wholesome approach to eating also grounds and calms the mind,
benefiting all three doshas.

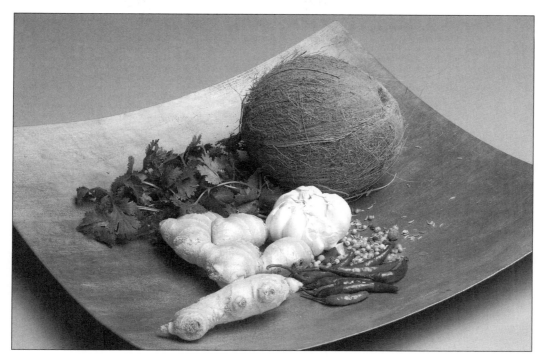

Ayurvedic cooking uses fresh herbs and spices that are both delicious and medicinal.

6. Have proper cooking tools on hand.

In India, the majority of Ayurvedic cooking is done with a few simple pots and pans. Some tools that are helpful for more advanced recipes are the following.

stainless steel soup pot and lid	pressure cooker
medium-sized frying pan and lid	mortar and pestle
heavy cast-iron frying pan	or coffee grinder (for
blender or food processor	grinding spices)

7. Create a sattvic atmosphere.

The intention and energy within a kitchen is an important invisible ingredient to the food we consume. You can establish a calm, pleasant atmosphere by bringing your full attention to what you are doing and proceeding with patience, care, and love. You may want to play harmonious music or recite a chant as you cook. In many traditions, a small sacred space is created in the kitchen where a small portion of the meal is offered to the divine spirit.

Food absorbs the vibrations created during the preparation of the meal, which then enter our bodies during the digestion process. The quality of the food is greatly enhanced by loving attention—from how the vegetables are cut to how the spices are ground and carefully added. What results is a *prasad,* a holy offering to the divine.

SATTVIC, RAJASIC, AND TAMASIC DIETS

SATTVIC DIET 	Consists of a vegetarian diet of fresh organic fruits and vegetables, whole grains, and dairy products such as milk and ghee (clarified butter). Sattvic foods keep the body lean and agile and promote a calm, clear, and compassionate mind. Fresh buttermilk and easily digestible legumes, such as mung dal and lentils, are examples of sattvic food. While a mild sweet taste is considered sattvic, a strong sweet taste and stimulating spices such as cayenne, garlic, and asafoetida are avoided. This is the diet followed by yogis and is often offered at ashrams and meditation centers.
RAJASIC DIET 	Consists of food that is spicy, salty, and sour in taste. Vegetables such as onions or garlic and spicy and sour preparations such as ketchup and vinegar have rajasic qualities. Wines, pickles, and meat (particularly red meats) are rajasic in nature. Stimulating drinks such as coffee and tea, carbonated beverages, and all types of alcoholic drinks are also rajasic. These foods increase restlessness, anger, and irritability.
TAMASIC DIET 	Consists of stale, overheated, oily, and heavy foods and canned meat and fish products containing a lot of preservatives. These foods increase lethargy, ignorance, and apathy. Frozen and preserved foods as well as genetically modified foods also increase the tamasic quality.

Much of our daily life revolves around nourishing ourselves by making appropriate choices as we shop for food and then cook, eat, and digest it. The more mindful we are in carrying out these activities, the more we are capable of optimizing the nutritional value that we derive from our food, thereby enhancing our health and well-being. As we become aware of our doshic type, it becomes possible to increase the healing quality surrounding each of these activities. As we will see in the next chapter, this brings us closer to integrating Ayurveda for life.

Ayurveda for Life

The word *ayurveda* is often translated as "the knowledge of our daily living"; in other words, Ayurveda concerns our lifestyle. Everything we think, do, see, and feel affects our constitutional makeup, moving the doshas in one way or another. The choices that we make on a daily basis have the ability to balance or disrupt our natural constitution. Over time these decisions affect our overall health, as the continuous repetition of an action gives it power. Whether it is a chosen career path, leisure activities, habits, or daily routines of sleep and exercise, each lifestyle choice that we make has the power to create harmony or discord in our lives.

When a person visits an Ayurvedic physician or consultant, a great deal of time is spent on questions that monitor every aspect of daily living. This helps the patient and the practitioner to ferret out the root cause of a particular heath problem. Rather than masking symptoms with the use of unnecessary and sometimes dangerous pharmaceuticals, Ayurveda teaches us to discover the root cause of the problem. As a result, the path of healing presented by Ayurveda is long-term and lasting, and encourages people to take responsibility for their own health.

During this age of media overload and hypermobility, the vata dosha within each of us is particularly prone to disturbance, causing nervousness, anxiety, depression, insomnia, and fear. It is estimated that a vast majority of all diseases are triggered by the body's reaction to stress. The Western medical community now widely recognizes the importance of preventive measures such as exercise, diet, and lifestyle in helping reduce the negative effects of stress on the body and mind.

At a certain intuitive level we all know what is good for us—yet the vast majority of people do not listen to the body when making lifestyle choices. For example, most of us know that excessive alcohol consumption is likely to cause a hangover or emotional disturbances the following day. Yet many people continue to use alcohol as a means of releasing stress, and then find themselves needing to use aspirin or caffeine to counteract the side effects. In this stress-reduction cycle the symptoms of a problem are masked, leaving the root cause actively brewing under the surface. After a time the body cannot handle this accumulation of stress and so begins to malfunction, sowing the seeds of disease and ill health.

Throughout the Ayurvedic classical texts is a common message reverberating the Buddhist concept of the middle way. The key to health and happiness is moderation—whether it be in food, exercise, sleep, sex, or work. In Ayurveda, right living does not necessitate following rigid rules; instead it means taking responsibility for our choices and acknowledging the consequences of our daily actions. As Dr. Jivaka Kumarbhaccha demonstrated during his final exam before becoming an Ayurvedic physician, everything around us can and should be used for healing purposes. Although we may not be able to implement every lifestyle tip recommended for our dosha, we can gradually attune our daily activities to flow with our natural constitution.

The table on pages 187 to 189 provides a summary of the most crucial lifestyle tips corresponding to each dosha, many of which we have touched on in previous chapters. These maintenance therapies provide a straightforward guide for practitioners and recipients to follow on a regular basis in order to take control of their own health and well-being.

THE WELLNESS THERAPY PROGRAM

This last part of the book has introduced three main components that can be combined to form a customized post-massage follow up—yoga postures and approach, Ayurvedic nutrition guidelines, and lifestyle tips. In our work with clients we integrate these components in a five-session process, during which we progressively introduce the recommendations and note them in the client file for follow up at the next session. We have reproduced this form for you in the appendix; see pages 198 to 200.

The key to this Wellness Therapy Program is to introduce Ayurveda into the lives of our clients in a gradual and nonintrusive way that invites individuals to establish their own long-term wellness goals. The Wellness Therapy form on pages 198 to 200 provides a structure that enables the practitioner to follow up on recommendations from the previous session and maintain a progress record. Through this approach practitioners have an opportunity to get to know their clients at a deeper level and over time.

LIFESTYLE TIPS FOR VATA

	VATA DOSHA
Atmosphere	Avoid too much noise, excessive talking or thinking, distraction, over-activity, overstimulation through the media, and a highly scheduled life. A secure and stable lifestyle that breeds happiness, joy, and contentment is best.
Weather/temperature	Avoid wind and extreme cold—warm, cozy environments are best.
Seasons	Vata seasons are fall and winter, so take particular care to follow a vata-balancing diet and routine during these times.
Colors	Warming colors such as red, orange, gold, and yellow diluted with moist colors, such as white, are best. Avoid loud and contrasting colors.
Hobbies	Self-care routines such as yoga, meditation, and massage are recommended. Excess traveling can drain vata energy and cause disharmony.
Sleep	Allow for plenty of physical rest and mental relaxation. Take naps during the day as needed and avoid staying up late. Make sure to have a soft and comfortable bed.
Routine	Vata types do best with regularity and routine in diet, activities, and sleep.
Work environment	Vatas perform best in a job with a low level of strenuous physical activity, with frequent breaks, and without close scrutiny and pressure. Excessively long hours are difficult for vatas, as are extremely competitive and demanding fields of work. Vatas need to find work that embraces their creativity and communication skills. Vatas excel as artists, dancers, musicians, writers, philosophers, computer programmers, journalists, and filmmakers.
Relationships	Primary relationships should be secure and nurturing, without too much volatility or conflict. Vatas are easily hurt and can be drawn into over-analyzing problems. Avoid this tendency; focus on positive and loving thoughts instead.
Exercise	Mild exercise such as gentle yoga, tai chi, and swimming are recommended. Avoid strong physical exertion, such as running or aerobics.
Hydrotherapy	Steam baths, salt or mineral baths, and hot tubs are good (do not stay in too long) followed by plenty of liquid intake and rest.

LIFESTYLE TIPS FOR PITTA

 PITTA DOSHA

Atmosphere	Avoid conflict, argument, aggression, ambition, too much strain, and competitive environments. Practice sweetness of speech, forgiveness, and contentment.
Weather/temperature	Cool breezes and moonlight are best. Avoid sun, heat, and torrid climates.
Seasons	Pitta seasons are late spring and summer, so take particular care to follow a pitta-balancing diet and routine during these times.
Colors	Cool colors such as blue, green, white, and pastels are best. Avoid too many hot and stimulating colors.
Hobbies	Relaxation, diversion, amusement, and play are recommended, as are noncompetitive sports, gardening, and water activities.
Sleep	Pittas should go to sleep before 10 PM to avoid restlessness in the night.
Routine	Moderate routine and regularity in diet, sleep, and activities help to keep pitta calm and cool, although they may find this annoying or difficult at first!
Work environment	Pittas should search for a pleasant work atmosphere that challenges the intellect without being overly competitive. Pittas tend to be workaholics; they need to make time for activities outside of work, such as family, relationships, and hobbies. Pittas excel as scientists, engineers, teachers, lawyers, business professionals, researchers, psychologists, orators, police officers, and politicians.
Relationships	Pittas' primary relationships should be calming, noncompetitive, and loving with plenty of affection and joy. Pittas tend to react with anger and control, and should avoid getting stuck in long, drawn-out arguments and debates.
Exercise	The best exercise for pitta is moderate exercise in the cool air and wind, or walking at night, especially under the moon. Strong aerobic exercise or heavy exertion should be avoided, especially under the sun. Exercise should not cause strong perspiration.
Hydrotherapy	Take cooling showers or baths, avoid hot tubs and saunas.

LIFESTYLE TIPS FOR KAPHA

	KAPHA DOSHA
Atmosphere	Awaken the mind and senses to break up stagnation and inactivity. Break attachments and habits, giving up unnecessary possessions and indulgences.
Weather/temperature	A dry and warm environment is best; avoid dampness and cold. Exposure to dry heat, sun, fire, and warm breezes is recommended.
Seasons	Kapha seasons are late winter and spring, so take particular care to follow a kapha-balancing diet and routine during these times.
Colors	Warm, dry, and stimulating colors such as red, orange, and yellow benefit kapha. Avoid white and cooling colors.
Hobbies	It is good for kaphas to engage in physical work and effort, as well as camping and taking long hikes. Gardening, singing, travel, charity work, devotion, and cooking for others are all beneficial.
Sleep	An austere sleeping environment, such as camping or sleeping on the floor, is good for kaphas. Avoid sleeping for long periods and during the day.
Routine	Too much routine is not advisable for kaphas. Stay up late, take a trip, or take on a new project in order to break the routine every once in a while.
Work environment	Kaphas excel at bringing things into form and creating institutions or establishments. Due to their strong interpersonal skills, kaphas make good managers, parents, providers, singers, real estate agents, and bankers. Discipline, some physical exertion, and mental stimulation are recommended.
Relationships	Primary relationships should be encouraging, stimulating, and supportive. Kaphas can be overly sentimental and possessive and therefore thrive in relationships that encourage loving space and compassionate support.
Exercise	Stimulating aerobic exercise in the wind and sun is recommended, as long as the individual is adequately strong and healthy. Hot and invigorating yoga and heavy physical activity, such as gardening or construction, can be beneficial. Exercise should raise a strong sweat and leave one feeling tired, but not exhausted.
Hydrotherapy	Strong sweating therapies that use dry heat, such as saunas, are recommended.

Such an exchange is rewarding for practitioners, who are able to see the long-term positive effects of the Ayurveda and Thai Yoga Therapy.

The first step in applying Thai Yoga Therapy in relationship with a client is to determine the client's Ayurvedic constitution using the Ayurvedic consultation form and Ayurvedic constitutional test provided in the appendix. Before attempting to understand the Ayurvedic dosha of others, though, we must identify our own constitution and work toward living in harmony with our own nature. It is only by living an Ayurvedic lifestyle that we can truly integrate this profound science into our bodywork practice.

When working with a client the practitioner should fill out the constitutional test for the recipient, to allow for more thorough analysis and exchange. The process of discovering one's Ayurvedic constitution is akin to holding a mirror in front your face; many recipients may feel uncomfortable with what they see. It is therefore important to be tactful and sensitive in our approach and to avoid pressing recipients to answer any question that may make them feel uncomfortable.

Just as with any professional counseling session, begin your first session by letting your client know that all information is kept strictly confidential. The best time to complete an assessment is during a prearranged thirty-minute period before a regular massage session.

Our success as conduits of Ayurveda is not dependent upon how much knowledge we can impress our client with, but with how effective we are in getting them to take responsibility for their own health. In this way Ayurveda encourages recipients to play an active role in their own healing process instead of simply passively receiving treatments. An important aspect of Ayurvedic counseling is to help our recipients set long-term self-care goals. However, we must allow these changes to come from them and avoid lecturing or being judgmental. Remain neutral yet supportive, embodying compassion and metta. Free treatment is not usually as effective, so make sure that you receive fair compensation or an exchange for your services.

Before completing the Ayurvedic constitutional test there are a few key points to keep in mind. It is important to remember that vata, pitta, and kapha are separate aspects of the same energy and are therefore always present in a living being. Vata individuals must have a certain proportion of the other doshas in order to exist; the same applies for the other constitutional types. You are therefore bound to have checks in all three columns of the constitutional test form.

As we mentioned earlier, a person's constitution remains the same throughout his or her life. It helps to observe the attributes revealed during your entire lifetime, not just in the past few months or years. It also helps to observe yourself in relationship to those around you for a better understanding of your doshic qualities. If you fall equally between two responses, check both columns. You may also leave blank any questions that are too difficult to answer.

Several attributes stand out as key indicators in the identification of doshic constitution. Physical attributes that tend to remain constant throughout a person's lifetime are important indicators—attributes such as body frame, height, weight, and complexion. It is also useful to note whether a person tends to be especially cold, which may indicate vata, or is especially hot, which could indicate pitta. Finally, pay close attention to a person's digestive and metabolic tendencies, which tend to reveal doshic imbalances. A person who has constipation or gas is more likely to have high vata, while acid stomach or heartburn points to excessive pitta. Kapha individuals often have a slow metabolism, which can cause bloating, mucus, or a sluggish digestion when aggravated. These points should give you good guidance in helping determine your own dosha and that of your clients.

We hope that you have enjoyed this voyage together with us through the ancient arts of Ayurveda and Thai Yoga Massage, and the blending of the two that we have created in developing Thai Yoga Therapy. In our parting words, we would like to reflect on the wisdom of the ancient Vedic texts that remind us that all knowledge is self-knowledge. Before we can begin helping others to achieve harmony and well-being, we must first cultivate those healing qualities in ourselves. Wherever you are on your path, may you walk in peace, self-knowledge, and compassion.

Appendices

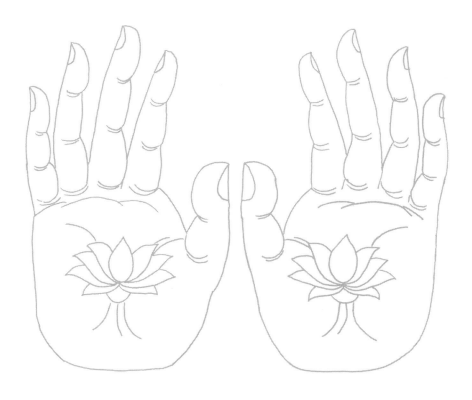

AYURVEDIC CONSULTATION FORM

Name: _____ Date: ___/___/___

Address: _____

Phone (home): (____) ____ _____   Phone (work): (____) ____ _____

Date of birth: ___/___/___   Occupation: _____

Major surgeries / conditions / medication:

Common ailments experienced by the client:

Regular exercise habits:

General eating and drinking habits:

Main purpose for visit:

AYURVEDIC CONSTITUTIONAL TEST
(MARK ONE OR MORE COLUMNS PER QUESTION)

		VATA		PITTA		KAPHA
Frame		Thin, light physique		Medium, developed physique		Stocky, big, thick, well-developed physique
Height		Exceptionally tall or short		Average		Tall and sturdy or short and stocky
Weight		Low weight; prominent veins and bones		Moderate weight; good muscles		Heavy; tends toward being overweight
Skin		Dry, rough, cold, dull, dark, tans easily, cracked		Red, glowing, soft, moist, warm; moles and freckles; tendency toward acne and sunburn		Fair, pale, thick, soft, smooth, moist, and cool
Hair		Dry, wiry, scanty, coarse, dandruff Color tendency: brown, black		Moderate, fine, soft, early baldness or grey Color tendency: light colors, red		Abundant, oily, soft, lustrous, thick, wavy Color tendency: light or dark
Face		Small features; thin, delicate, long structure; early wrinkles		Sharp features; angular structure; reddish; forehead folds		Large, round features
Eyes		Small, dry, unsteady, dark, dull; small eyelashes		Medium, piercing, easily inflamed (red), sensitive to light, light colors		Wide, white, attractive; long eyelashes; calm
Lips		Thin, small, dry, cracked; may tremble		Medium, soft, red		Large, moist, smooth, firm
Teeth		Thin, small, tend to be crooked; spaces between teeth; receding gums		Medium size; yellowish; bleeding gums		Large, thick, white

		VATA	PITTA	KAPHA
Chest		Thin, narrow, flat, underdeveloped	Medium development	Broad, large, well developed
Hands		Small, narrow; dry, cold, rough; pronounced veins or knuckles; may tremble	Medium, reddish; moist; warm	Large, thick, oily; cool; square or round shape
Nails		Small, thin, dry, rough, cracked, brittle	Medium, soft, pink	Large, thick, smooth, white, firm
Feet		Small, narrow, long, dry, rough	Medium, soft, pink	Large, thick, wide
Voice		Low, weak, hoarse, rapid, talkative, unfocused	High-pitched, sharp, moderate, convincing, argumentative	Pleasant, deep, good tone, slow, not talkative
Sleep		Light; tends toward insomnia	Moderate; may wake up but will fall back to sleep	Heavy; difficult to wake up
Urine		Scanty, difficult, colorless; may be foamy	Profuse, yellow, red, burning	Moderate, may be whitish or milky
Feces		Scanty, dry, hard; tends toward constipation and gas	Abundant, loose, yellowish; tends toward diarrhea with burning sensation	Moderate, slow, solid; may have mucous
Sweat		Scanty, variable, odorless	Profuse, hot, strong smell	Moderate, cold
Appetite		Variable, insufficient	Strong; not able to skip meals	Constant but low; may use food as an escape
Thirst		Variable	Excessive	Scanty, little
Circulation		Poor, variable	Good, warm	Slow, steady
Activity		Hyperactive; quick, fast, erratic	Medium; motivated, purposeful, goal seeking	Slow, steady, could be lethargic

		VATA		PITTA		KAPHA
Sensitivity		Cold, wind, dryness		Heat, sun, fire		Cold, damp
Strength/ endurance		Poor, variable, starts and stops quickly		Medium, intolerant of heat		Strong, slow to start but good endurance
Disease tendency		Nervous-system issues, pain, arthritis, mental disorders, emaciation, insomnia		Fevers, infections, inflammatory diseases		Respiratory-system disease, congestion, mucous, water retention
Neurotic tendencies		Anxiety attacks, trembling		Temper, rage, hot-headed tantrums		Deep sorrow, stagnation
Mental nature— positive		Active, adaptable, creative, enthusiastic		Intelligent, precise, competitive, articulate, focused		Calm, stable, content, patient, affectionate, down-to-earth
Mental nature— negative		Indecisive, fearful, anxious, nervous, "worry-wart," over-sensitive		Aggressive, irritable, tendency toward anger and frustration		Slow to change, can be lazy, overly attached and sentimental
Totals		_____ Vata		_____ Pitta		_____ Kapha

Predominant dosha(s): _____

WELLNESS THERAPY PROGRAM

Client name: _____

Predominant dosha(s): _____   Doshic ratio: _____(V) _____(P) _____(K)

Main purpose for visit: _____

❖

1ST SESSION: CUSTOMIZED AYURVEDA AND
THAI YOGA THERAPY SESSION

Date: ___/___/____

Recipient's general reaction to massage: _____

_____

Contraindications encountered: _____

2ND SESSION: CUSTOMIZED SESSION WITH
BASIC YOGA RECOMMENDATIONS

Date:___/___/____

Recipient's general reaction to massage: _____

_____

Contraindications encountered: _____

Yoga practice recommendations: _____

_____

3RD SESSION: CUSTOMIZED SESSION
WITH BASIC NUTRITIONAL RECOMMENDATIONS

Date:___/___/____

Recipient's general reaction to massage: _____

Contraindications encountered: _____

Yoga practice follow up:_____

_____

Basic nutritional recommendations: _____

_____

4TH SESSION: CUSTOMIZED SESSION AND
LIFESTYLE RECOMMENDATIONS

Date:___/___/____

Recipient's general reaction to massage: _____

_____

Contraindications encountered: _____

Nutritional recommendations follow up:_____

_____

Lifestyle recommendations:_____

_____

5TH SESSION: CUSTOMIZED SESSION AND
LONG-TERM AYURVEDIC GOALS

Date:___/___/____

Recipient's general reaction to massage: _____

_____

Contraindications encountered: _____

Lifestyle recommendations:_____

_____

Long-term self-care Ayurvedic goals:

_____

_____

_____

_____

Thai Yoga Therapy
Sequence for Vatas

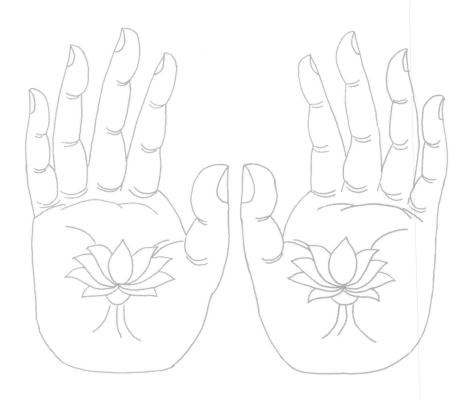

Namaskar (p. 87)

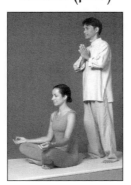

Palming Shoulders (p. 88)

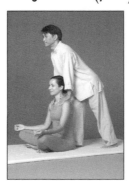

Whirlpool (p. 94)

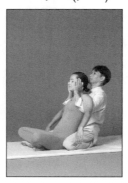

Forward Bend (p. 98)

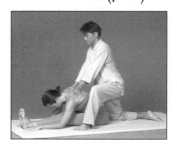

Foot Sandwich (p. 104)

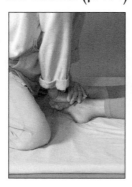

Kneeing Insteps (p. 105)

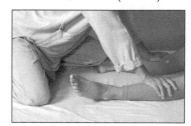

Mortar and Pestle (p. 107)

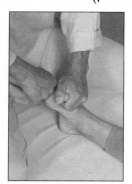

Shoe Polish (p. 108)

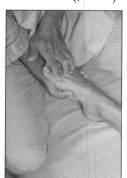

Palming Sen on Medial Side (p. 111)

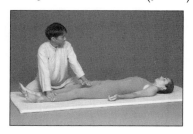

Helicopter (p. 113)

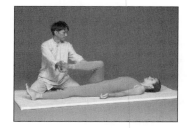

Demi Lotus (p. 118)

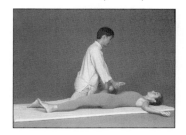

Demi Diamond (p. 119)

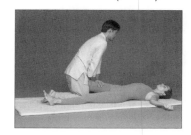

Sole Roll (p. 123)

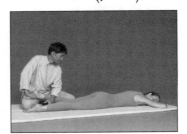

Frog (p. 125)

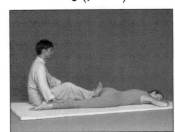

Reverse Lotus (p. 126)

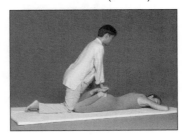

Palming Back (p. 127)

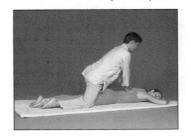

Pillow Cobra (p. 129)

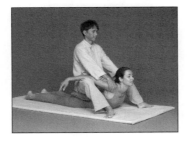

Crescent Moon (p. 133)

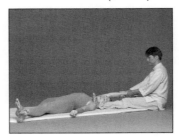

Tortoise (p. 135)

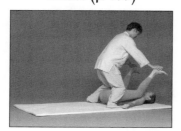

Thai Lute (p. 137)

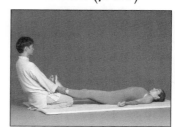

Lay-a-Brick (p. 139)

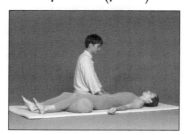

Sun-Moon Stroke (p. 140)

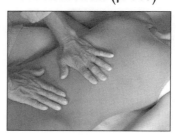

Massaging the Organ-
Reflex Points (p. 141)

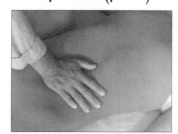

Finger Pressing (p. 142)

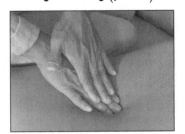

Opening the Chest (p. 143)

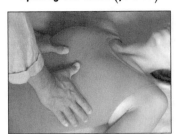

Palming Arms (p. 144)

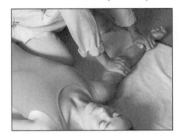

Hand Massage (p. 145)

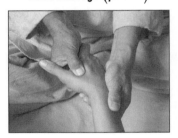

Marma Face Massage (p. 147)

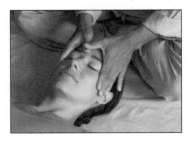

Thai Yoga Therapy
Sequence for Pittas

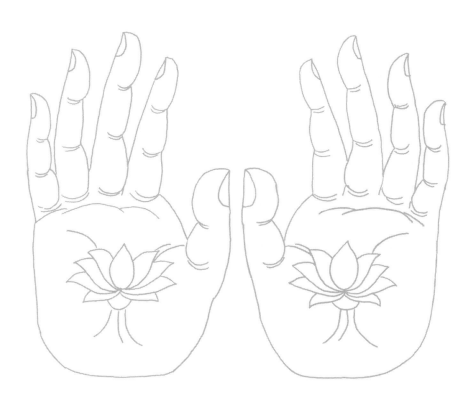

Namaskar (p. 87)

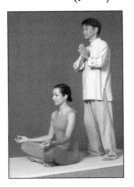

Palming Shoulders (p. 88)

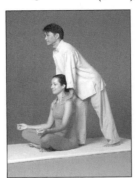

Lunar Stretch (p. 91)

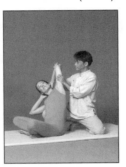

Shakti Twist (p. 93)

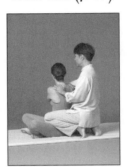

Forward Bend (p. 98)

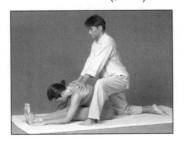

Amsa Pressure (p. 102)

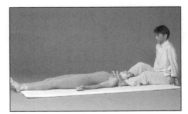

Foot Sandwich (p. 104)

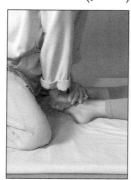

Kneeing Insteps (p. 105)

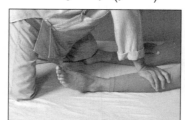

Mortar and Pestle (p. 107)

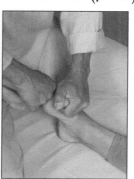

Shoe Polish (p. 108)

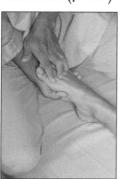

Toe Dance (p. 109)

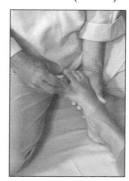

**Palming Sen on
Medial Side (p. 111)**

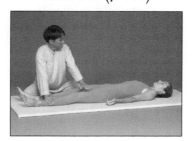

**Helicopter
(p. 113)**

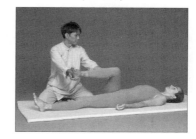

Nataraj (p. 114)

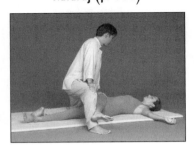

Hugging Tree (p. 116)

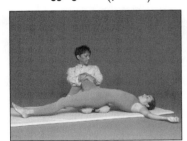

Demi Lotus (p. 118)

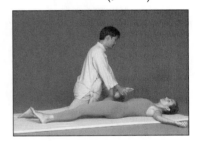

Demi Diamond (p. 119)

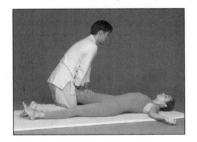

Sole Roll (p. 123)

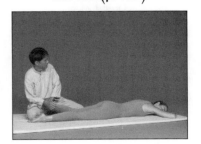

Reverse Lotus (p. 126)

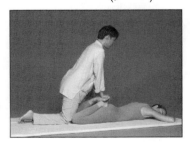

Palming Back (p. 127)

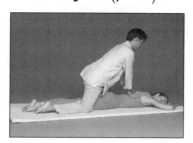

Classical Cobra (p. 130)

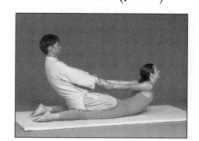

Crescent Moon (p. 133)

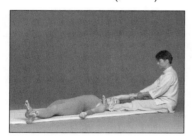

Tortoise (p. 135)

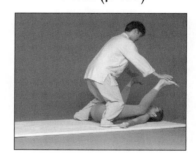

Hip Swirl (p. 136)

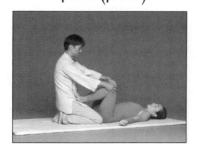

Thai Lute (p. 137)

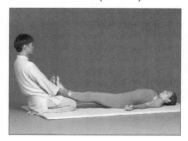

Lay-a-Brick (p. 139)

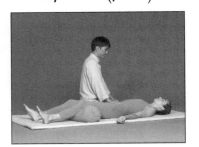

Sun-Moon Stroke (p. 140)

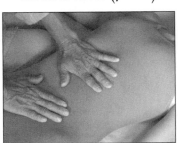

Massaging the Organ-Reflex Points (p. 141)

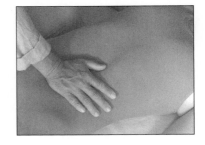

Finger Pressing (p. 142)

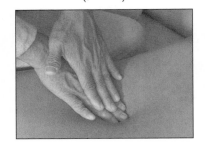

Palming Arms (p. 144)

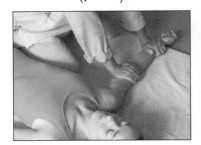

Hand Massage (p. 145)

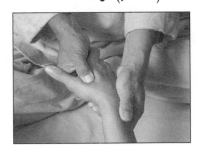

Marma Face Massage (p. 147)

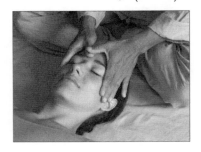

Thai Yoga Therapy Sequence for Kaphas

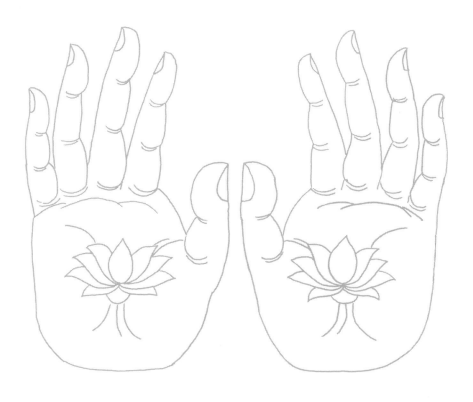

Namaskar (p. 87)

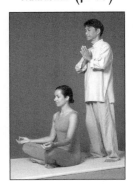

Udana Stretch (p. 89)

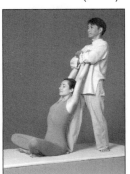

Butterfly Knee (p. 90)

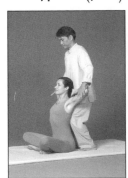

Lunar Stretch (p. 91)

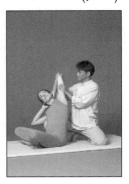

Shiva Twist (p. 92)

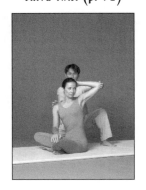

Shakti Twist (p. 93)

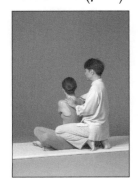

Bridge (p. 96)

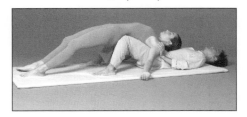

Fish (p. 99)

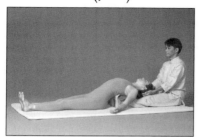

Counter Fish (p. 101)

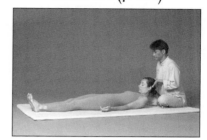

Amsa Pressure (p. 102)

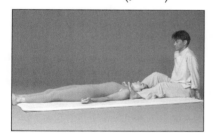

Foot Sandwich (p. 104)

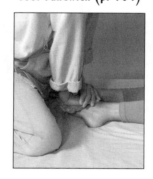

Kneeing Insteps (p. 105)

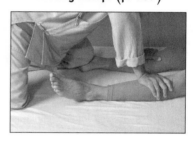

Toe Arc (p. 106)

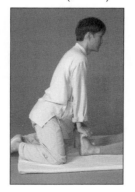

Toe Dance (p. 109)

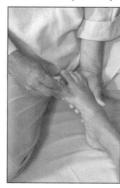

Palming Sen on Medial Side (p. 111)

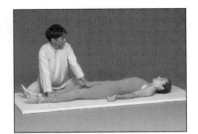

Kneeing Sen on Lateral Side (p. 112)

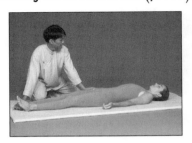

Helicopter (p. 113)

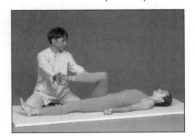

Nataraj (p. 114)

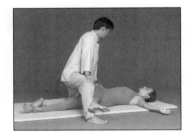

Stringing Bow (p. 115)

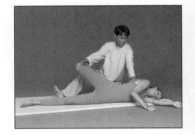

Hugging Tree (p. 116)

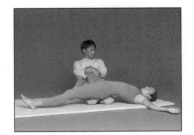

Demi Lotus (p. 118)

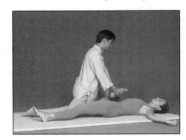

Demi Diamond (p. 119)

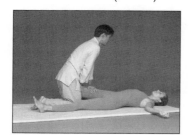

Janu Pump (p. 124)

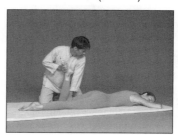

Frog (p. 125)

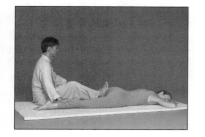

Reverse Lotus (p. 126)

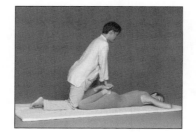

Kneeing Back (p. 128)

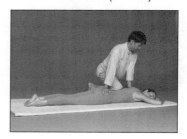

Classical Cobra (p. 130)

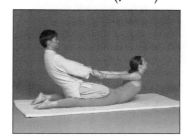

Crescent Moon (p. 133)

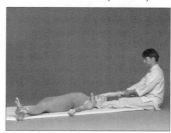

Tea Pot (p. 134)

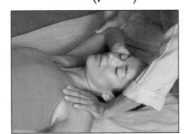

Tortoise (p. 135)

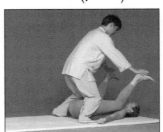

Hip Swirl (p. 136)

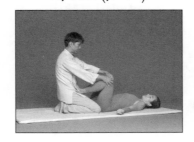

Sun-Moon Stroke (p. 140)

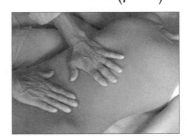

Opening the Chest (p. 143)

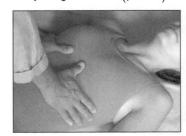

Palming Arms (p. 144)

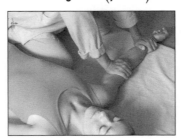

Marma Face Massage (p. 147)

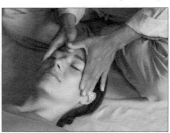

Resources

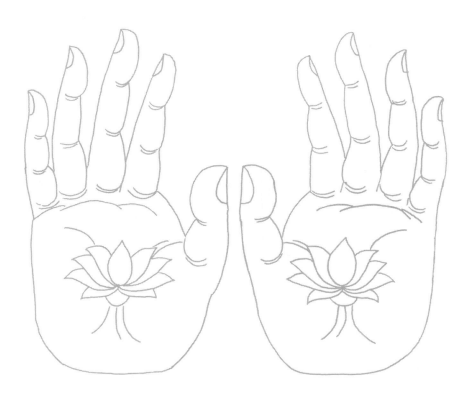

THAI YOGA MASSAGE TRAINING

The Lotus Palm School, founded by Kam Thye Chow, is one of the first Thai Yoga Massage schools in North America to have our certification program recognized for practice as a base modality by professional massage associations, including the National Certification Board for Therapeutic Massage and Bodywork (NCBTMB) and Fédération Québécoise des Massothérapeutes (FQM).

Our instructors teach courses worldwide. Please consult our website for the most up-to-date teaching schedule. If you are interested in hosting Lotus Palm for a workshop in your area, please be in touch.

> Lotus Palm School of Thai Yoga Massage
> 5337 St. Laurent, Suite 240
> Montreal, Quebec
> Canada H2T 1S5
> www.lotuspalm.com
> info@lotuspalm.com

PRACTICE AIDS

The Lotus Palm School offers a complete product line of Thai Yoga Massage items to support and inspire your practice.

Lotus Palm Mat Set

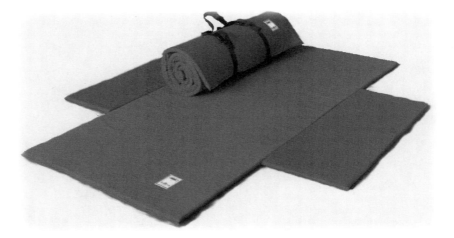

The Lotus Palm mat set consists of the main mat and two portable side mats, enabling the practitioner to expand the width of the mat and offering easy access to the removable mats from either side. These mats are suitable for Thai massage, shiatsu, Phoenix Rising yoga therapy, Breema, and all forms of floor work.

Mat specifications

- Each mat is made of dense compressed foam
- 100% high-quality, durable cotton cover
- 3 strong nylon carrying straps, 2" wide, with buckle
- Under 20 lbs.
- Color: Burgundy
- Size: 1 main mat (83" x 39" x 1") and 2 side mats (16" x 39" x 1")

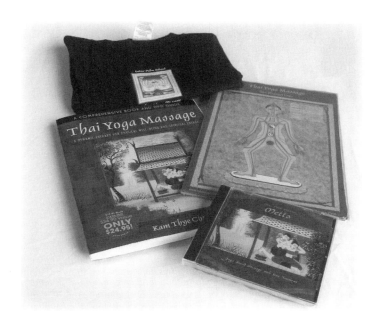

Other Products

Thai Yoga Massage book and DVD by Kam Thye Chow
Lotus Palm Music CD by Uwe Neumann
Handmade Thai Pants specifically for bodywork
Sheets for the massage mat
Pillows for massage and prenatal Thai Massage
T-shirts
Meditation cushions

To order mats, books, DVDs, CDs, clothes, meditation cushions, and sheets:
1-800-585-5713
www.lotuspalm.com

BOOKS OF RELATED INTEREST

Thai Yoga Massage
A Dynamic Therapy for Physical Well-Being and
Spiritual Energy
Book & DVD Set
by Kam Thye Chow

The Handbook of Chinese Massage
Tui Na Techniques to Awaken Body and Mind
by Maria Mercati

Trigger Point Therapy for Myofascial Pain
The Practice of Informed Touch
*by Donna Finando, L.Ac., L.M.T., and
Steven Finando, Ph.D., L.Ac.*

Rolfing
Reestablishing the Natural Alignment and
Structural Integration of the Human Body for
Vitality and Well-Being
by Ida P. Rolf, Ph.D.

Amma Therapy
A Complete Textbook of Oriental Bodywork and
Medical Principles
by Tina Sohn and Robert Sohn

The Reflexology Atlas
*by Bernard C. Kolster, M.D. and
Astrid Waskowiak, M.D.*

The Heart of Yoga
Developing a Personal Practice
by T. K. V. Desikachar

Applied Kinesiology
Muscle Response in Diagnosis, Therapy, and
Preventive Medicine
by Tom and Carole Valentine with Douglas P. Hetrick, D.C.

Inner Traditions • Bear & Company
P.O. Box 388
Rochester, VT 05767
1-800-246-8648
www.InnerTraditions.com

Or contact your local bookseller